T0259406

Collaborative Antimicrobial Stewardship

Editors

ELIZABETH DODDS ASHLEY
STEVEN SCHAEFFER SPIRES

INFECTIOUS DISEASE CLINICS
OF NORTH AMERICA

www.id.theclinics.com

Consulting Editor
HELEN W. BOUCHER

March 2020 • Volume 34 • Number 1

ELSEVIER

1600 John F. Kennedy Boulevard ● Suite 1800 ● Philadelphia, Pennsylvania, 19103-2899.

http://www.theclinics.com

INFECTIOUS DISEASE CLINICS OF NORTH AMERICA Volume 34, Number 1
March 2020 ISSN 0891–5520, ISBN-13: 978-0-323-68393-7

Editor: Kerry Holland
Developmental Editor: Donald Mumford

Infectious Disease Clinics of North America (ISSN 0891–5520) is published in March, June, September, and December by Elsevier Inc., 360 Park Avenue South, New York, NY 10010-1710. Periodicals postage paid at New York, NY and additional mailing offices. Subscription prices are $340.00 per year for US individuals, $703.00 per year for US institutions, $100.00 per year for US students, $396.00 per year for Canadian individuals, $878.00 per year for Canadian institutions, $432.00 per year for international individuals, $878.00 per year for international institutions, $100.00 per year for Canadian students, and $200.00 per year for international students. To receive student rate, orders must be accompanied by name of affiliated institution, date of term, and the *signature* of program/residency coordinator on institution letterhead. Orders will be billed at individual rate until proof of status is received. Foreign air speed delivery is included in all *Clinics* subscription prices. All prices are subject to change without notice. **POSTMASTER**: Send address changes to *Infectious Disease Clinics of North America*, Elsevier Health Sciences Division, Subcription Customer Service, 3251 Riverport Lane, Maryland Heights, MO 63043. **Customer Service: 1-800-654-2452 (US). From outside of the US and Canada, call 1-314-447-8871. Fax: 1-314-447-8029. E-mail: JournalsCustomerService-usa@elsevier.com (print support) or JournalsOnlineSupport-usa@elsevier.com (online support).**

Infectious Disease Clinics of North America is also published in Spanish by Editorial Inter-Médica, Junin 917, 1er A 1113, Buenos Aires, Argentina.

Reprints. For copies of 100 or more, of articles in this publication, please contact the Commercial Reprints Department, Elsevier Inc., 360 Park Avenue South, New York, New York 10010-1710. Tel. 212-633-3874, Fax: 212-633-3820, E-mail: reprints@elsevier.com.

Infectious Disease Clinics of North America is covered in *MEDLINE/PubMed (Index Medicus), Current Contents/ Clinical Medicine, Science Citation Alert, SCISEARCH,* and *Research Alert.*

Contributors

CONSULTING EDITOR

HELEN W. BOUCHER, MD, FIDSA, FACP
Director, Infectious Diseases Fellowship Program, Division of Geographic Medicine and Infectious Diseases, Tufts Medical Center, Associate Professor of Medicine, Tufts University School of Medicine, Boston, Massachusetts

EDITORS

ELIZABETH DODDS ASHLEY, PharmD, MHS, FCCP, BCPS
Associate Professor of Medicine, Duke Center for Antimicrobial Stewardship and Infection Prevention, Division of Infectious Diseases, Duke University School of Medicine, Durham, North Carolina

STEVEN SCHAEFFER SPIRES, MD
Assistant Professor of Medicine, Duke Center for Antimicrobial Stewardship and Infection Prevention, Division of Infectious Diseases, Duke University School of Medicine, Durham, North Carolina

AUTHORS

NICOLE M. ACQUISTO, PharmD
Emergency Medicine Clinical Pharmacy Specialist, Department of Pharmacy, Associate Professor, Department of Emergency Medicine, University of Rochester Medical Center, Rochester, New York

CULLEN ADRE, PharmD
Tennessee Department of Health, Nashville, Tennessee

ADAMO BRANCACCIO, PharmD
Department of Pharmacy Services, Michigan Medicine, University of Michigan, College of Pharmacy, Ann Arbor, Michigan

WHITNEY R. BUCKEL, PharmD
Intermountain Healthcare Pharmacy Services, Taylorsville, Utah

LISA E. DAVIDSON, MD
Medical Director, Antimicrobial Support Network, Associate Professor, Internal Medicine, Division of Infectious Diseases, Atrium Health, Charlotte, North Carolina

CHRISTOPHER D. EVANS, PharmD
Pharmacist, Tennessee Department of Health, Healthcare Associated Infections and Antimicrobial Resistance Program, Nashville, Tennessee

KRISTIN FISCHER, BM, MM
Research Analyst II, Department of Medicine, Division of Infectious Diseases, Atrium Health, Charlotte, North Carolina

ERIN M. GENTRY, PharmD, BCPS
Clinical Pharmacy Manager, Antimicrobial Support Network, Atrium Health, Charlotte, North Carolina

KEITH W. HAMILTON, MD
Associate Professor of Clinical Medicine, Perelman School of Medicine, Director of Antimicrobial Stewardship, Hospital of the University of Pennsylvania, Philadelphia, Pennsylvania

NICHOLAS BOWDITCH HAUSMAN, MBA
Consultant, Belmont, Massachusetts

ROBIN L.P. JUMP, MD, PhD
Geriatric Research Education and Clinical Center (GRECC), Specialty Care Center of Innovation at the VA Northeast Ohio Healthcare System, Division of Infectious Diseases and HIV Medicine, Departments of Medicine, and Population and Quantitative Health Sciences, Case Western Reserve University School of Medicine, Cleveland, Ohio

KEITH S. KAYE, MD, MPH
Division of Infectious Diseases, Department of Internal Medicine, University of Michigan, University of Michigan Medical School, Ann Arbor, Michigan

SHELLEY KESTER, MHA, BSN, RN, CIC
Assistant Vice President, Infection Prevention, Division of Quality, Atrium Health, Charlotte, North Carolina

KATHERINE KRAMME, DO
Surgery Resident, Department of Surgery, Western Michigan University Homer Stryker M.D. School of Medicine, Kalamazoo, Michigan

KRISTI M. KUPER, PharmD, BCPS
Director of Clinical Pharmacy, DoseMe/Tabula Rasa HealthCare, Moorestown, New Jersey

JAMES W. S. LEWIS, MD, MPH
Medical Epidemiologist Consultant, North Carolina Department of Health and Human Services, Division of Public Health, Communicable Disease Branch, Raleigh, North Carolina; Adjunct Assistant Professor of Epidemiology, UNC Gillings School of Global Public Health, Adjunct Assistant Professor of Medicine, UNC School of Medicine, Chapel Hill, North Carolina

MEGAN MACK, MD
Department of Internal Medicine, Michigan Medicine, University of Michigan, School of Medicine, Ann Arbor, Michigan

AMY J. MATHERS, MD, D(ABMM)
Associate Professor, Department of Medicine, Division of Infectious Diseases, University of Virginia, Charlottesville, Virginia

LARISSA MAY, MD, MSPH, MSHS
Professor and Director of Emergency Department and Outpatient Antibiotic Stewardship, Department of Emergency Medicine, UC Davis Health, Sacramento, California

JEROD NAGEL, PharmD
Department of Pharmacy Services, Michigan Medicine, University of Michigan, College of Pharmacy, Ann Arbor, Michigan

CHRISTOPHER A. OHL, MD
Department of Internal Medicine, Section on Infectious Diseases, Wake Forest Baptist
Health, Winston-Salem, North Carolina

RICHARD NEAL OLANS, MD, FIDSA
Director of Infectious Diseases and Antimicrobial Stewardship, Melrose Wakefield
Hospital, Melrose, Massachusetts

RITA DRUMMOND OLANS, DNP, RN, CPNP-PC, APRN-BC
Assistant Professor, School of Nursing, MGH Institute of Health Professions, Pediatric
Nurse Practitioner–Hospitalist, Spaulding Rehabilitation Hospital, Boston, Massachusetts

ELIZABETH L. PALAVECINO, MD
Department of Pathology, Wake Forest Baptist Health, Winston-Salem, North Carolina

CATHERINE L. PASSARETTI, MD
Medical Director, Health System Infection Prevention, Associate Professor, Internal
Medicine, Division of Infectious Diseases, Atrium Health, Charlotte, North Carolina

PAYAL K. PATEL, MD, MPH
Division of Infectious Diseases, Department of Internal Medicine, University of Michigan,
VA Ann Arbor Healthcare System, Ann Arbor, Michigan

KAYLA POPOVA, PharmD
Department of Pharmacy Services, Michigan Medicine, University of Michigan, College of
Pharmacy, Ann Arbor, Michigan

EVAN D. ROBINSON, MD
Infectious Diseases Fellow, Department of Medicine, Division of Infectious Diseases,
University of Virginia, Charlottesville, Virginia

ROBERT G. SAWYER, MD
Professor and Chair, Department of Surgery, Western Michigan University Homer Stryker
M.D. School of Medicine, Kalamazoo, Michigan

STEVEN SCHAEFFER SPIRES, MD
Assistant Professor of Medicine, Duke Center for Antimicrobial Stewardship and Infection
Prevention, Division of Infectious Diseases, Duke University School of Medicine, Durham,
North Carolina

DAVID F. VOLLES, Pharm D, BCCCP
Clinical Critical Care Pharmacist, Department of Pharmacy, University of Virginia,
Charlottesville, Virginia

JOHN C. WILLIAMSON, PharmD
Departments of Pharmacy and Internal Medicine, Section on Infectious Diseases, Wake
Forest Baptist Health, Winston-Salem, North Carolina

Contents

Successful antimicrobial stewardship programs rely on engagement with hospital administrators. Antimicrobial stewards should understand the unique pressures and demands of hospital and health system administration and be familiar with key terminology and regulatory requirements. This article provides guidance on strategies for engaging hospital and health system administration to support antimicrobial stewardship, including recommendations for designing a successful antimicrobial stewardship program structure, pitching resource requests, setting meaningful and measurable goals, achieving and communicating results, and fostering ongoing relationships with hospital and health system administration.

Overall goals of antibiotic stewardship and infection prevention programs are to improve patient safety as it pertains to risk of infection or multidrug-resistant organism (MDRO) acquisition. Although the focus of day-to-day activities may differ, the themes of surveillance, education, clinician engagement, and multidisciplinary interactions are prevalent in both programs. Synergistic work between programs has yielded benefits in prevention of MDROs, surgical site infections, *Clostridioides difficile* infection, and reducing inappropriate testing and treatment for asymptomatic bacteriuria. Collaboration between programs can help maximize resources and minimize redundant work to keep issues related to bugs and drugs at bay.

Information technology (IT) is vitally important to making antimicrobial stewardship a scalable endeavor in modern health care systems. Without IT, many antimicrobial interventions in patient care would be missed. Clinical decision support systems and smartphone apps, either stand-alone or integrated into electronic health records, can all be effective tools to help augment the work of antimicrobial stewardship programs and support the management of infectious diseases in any health care setting.

There have been tremendous advances in methodologies available for detection and identification of organisms causing infections. Providers can now obtain identification results and antimicrobial susceptibility results in a shorter period of time. However, declining health care resources highlight the importance of selecting the right test at the right time to maximize diagnostic benefits. Therefore, the role of the antimicrobial stewardship team in the clinical microbiology laboratory has expanded to include diagnostic stewardship and provision of guidance on test selection for diagnosis and management of infection. This review focuses on the experience of our group in collaborative stewardship, emphasizing successes and challenges.

Successful antimicrobial stewardship programs must be a truly collaborative multidisciplinary team effort. Nurses have critical contributions and are recognized more in publications about antimicrobial stewardship. Examination of patient care workflow patterns indicates the central role of nurses in the application of stewardship concepts in patient care. Education about antimicrobial resistance and antimicrobial stewardship is important not only for nurses and other health care providers but also for the general public. Analysis of the health care workforce population shows the importance of integrating this largest segment of health care providers in the routine daily care of patients into all stewardship efforts.

Hospitalists represent a rapidly emerging specialty group that treats a large proportion of hospitalized patients with infections. Antimicrobial stewardship programs and hospitalist groups that focus on building a collaborative approach have been extremely successful in optimizing antimicrobial prescribing and improving patient outcomes. We discuss the tools needed to build collaborative relationships, summarize published examples of successful stewardship-hospitalist collaboration, and provide guidance on developing collaborative interventions.

Antimicrobial stewardship efforts that include surgeons rely on healthy and open communications between surgeons, infectious diseases specialists, and pharmacists. These efforts most frequently are related to surgical prophylaxis, the management of surgical infections, and surgical critical care. Policy should be based on best evidence and timely interactions to develop consensus on how to develop appropriate guidelines and protocols. Flexibility on all sides leads to increasingly strong relationships over time.

Given the large number of patients seen in the emergency department (ED) and concerns with antibiotic overprescribing, the ED is an important setting to target for antimicrobial stewardship (AS) initiatives. The ED is positioned between ambulatory and inpatient settings, making AS collaboration with clinicians and other health care providers in the hospital, long-term care facilities, and ambulatory settings critical to success. This article details ED-focused AS strategies on empiric antimicrobial selection, prompt administration, preventing ED return and readmissions, suggested collaborations between ED AS leadership and other key partners, and potential future strategies for expansion.

Antimicrobial stewardship is a collaborative venture and antimicrobial stewardship in long-term care (LTC) settings is no exception. There are many barriers to implementing effective antimicrobial stewardship programs in LTC settings, including constrained financial resources, limited access to physicians and pharmacists with antimicrobial stewardship training, minimal on-site infectious syndrome diagnostics and laboratory expertise, and high rates of staff turnover. This article suggests that collaboration at the level of health care facilities and systems, with public health departments, with laboratory partners, and among personnel, including nursing staff, prescribers, and pharmacists, can lead to effective antimicrobial stewardship programs in LTC settings.

Given the population-level implications of antibiotic resistance and the importance of antibiotic stewardship in containment and prevention of resistance, public health has a vested interest in strengthening antibiotic stewardship efforts. There are opportunities for public health collaboration at all levels including local health departments, state public health programs, and through federal public health entities. This article discusses existing public health stewardship activities, opportunities for collaboration between public health and key partners in antibiotic stewardship programs, the potential for improvement and expansion of current activities, and possible new modes of collaboration that could be pursued.

INFECTIOUS DISEASE CLINICS OF NORTH AMERICA

THE CLINICS ARE AVAILABLE ONLINE!
Access your subscription at:
www.theclinics.com

Preface

Regarding Collaboration in Antimicrobial Stewardship

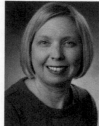

Elizabeth Dodds Ashley, PharmD, MHS, FCCP, BCPS   Steven Schaeffer Spires, MD
Editors

Clinicians were not meant to practice alone; instead, at best, medicine should be practiced as a team composed of multiple disciplines engendering a collective accountability for patient care. This type of practice highlights the strengths of individual health care professionals and depends on collaboration for success. Successful antimicrobial stewardship embodies this type of multidisciplinary collaboration, beginning with the combined leadership of a pharmacist and physician and drawing in the unique expertise and skillsets of each to build a team pulling from all areas in the health system involving antibiotic use. These key collaborations with nursing, laboratory, administration, and other physicians representing respective specialties comprise the exemplary antimicrobial stewardship program (ASP). In many cases, it is these collaborations that make the difference between successful and failing interventions and programs. These collaborations are the secret to stewardship success.

In this issue of *Infectious Disease Clinics of North America*, we aim to provide stories of how the challenges of developing effective ASPs are overcome by collaborating with partners in the hospital, including nursing, surgery, hospital medicine, emergency department, information technology, microbiology laboratory, infection prevention, and hospital administration. Also, partners outside the hospital are necessary in many settings and can have a larger impact on the community when public health departments, outpatient practices, and associated long-term care settings are involved. There are also reciprocal benefits for all when common interests are found and partnerships progress.

Antimicrobial stewardship, the optimization of the use of antimicrobials maximizing their benefits while minimizing the risks, is not something that is done to you or for you but has to be seen as something in which we all have a role to play. ASPs themselves cannot touch every patient receiving antimicrobials but require a partnership or functional relationship with those parties who do. Thus, effective collaboration is the hands

Infect Dis Clin N Am 34 (2020) xi–xii
https://doi.org/10.1016/j.idc.2019.12.001
0891-5520/20/© 2019 Published by Elsevier Inc.

and feet of antimicrobial stewardship. The authors in this issue were asked to write articles full of stories not only from the published literature but also from their own experience. We found these thoughtful reviews informative to our stewardship practice and are eager to share.

Elizabeth Dodds Ashley, PharmD, MHS, FCCP, BCPS
Duke Center for Antimicrobial Stewardship
and Infection Prevention
Division of Infectious Diseases
Duke University School of Medicine
Duke University Medical Center
PO Box 102359
Durham, NC 27710, USA

Steven Schaeffer Spires, MD
Duke Center for Antimicrobial Stewardship
and Infection Prevention
Division of Infectious Diseases
Duke University School of Medicine
Duke University Medical Center
PO Box 102359
Durham, NC 27710, USA

E-mail addresses:
Libby.dodds@duke.edu (E.D. Ashley)
Steven.spires@duke.edu (S.S. Spires)

Collaborative Antimicrobial Stewardship
Working with Hospital and Health System Administration

Whitney R. Buckel, PharmD[a],*, Keith S. Kaye, MD, MPH[b],
Payal K. Patel, MD, MPH[b,c]

KEYWORDS

- Antimicrobial stewardship • Antibiotic stewardship • Administration • Management
- C-suite

KEY POINTS

- Before interacting with hospital and health system administration, research local pressures, decision-making processes, key terminology, and regulatory requirements.
- When pitching resource requests, consider the regulatory, quality, and safety impacts of antimicrobial stewardship and think creatively for potential areas for improvement.
- When designing or redesigning the structure of an antimicrobial stewardship program within a hospital or health system, strongly consider aligning the reporting structure within the quality-of-care reporting lines.
- Foster ongoing relationships by being proactive in the goal-setting process, consistent in follow-through, and systematic and routine in communication.

INTRODUCTION

Successful antimicrobial stewardship programs (ASPs) rely on engagement by hospital administrators.[1,2] References to hospital administration traditionally describe the C-suite, including the chief executive officer, chief medical officer, and chief nursing officer. There are many additional positions that may compose the C-suite, such as chief quality officers and chief pharmacy officers. Structures differ across hospitals and health systems, and the relevant power and influence of each role also varies.

[a] Intermountain Healthcare Pharmacy Services, 4393 South Riverboat Road, Suite 100, Taylorsville, UT 84123, USA; [b] Division of Infectious Diseases, Department of Internal Medicine, University of Michigan, Ann Arbor, MI, USA; [c] Division of Infectious Diseases, Department of Internal Medicine, Veterans Affairs Ann Arbor Healthcare System, VA Ann Arbor Healthcare System (111-I), 2215 Fuller Road, Ann Arbor, MI 48109-2399, USA
* Corresponding author.
E-mail address: whitney.buckel@imail.org

Infect Dis Clin N Am 34 (2020) 1–15
https://doi.org/10.1016/j.idc.2019.10.003
0891-5520/20/© 2019 Elsevier Inc. All rights reserved.

id.theclinics.com

In addition, the clinical background of the administrator and institution size also affect how the antimicrobial stewardship program interacts with administration. Understanding the unique dynamics of each individual setting, including who is responsible for decisions and how these decisions are made, can help antimicrobial stewardship to be successful. Although outside the scope of this review, it is valuable to consider other key stakeholders in leadership positions who can be advocates and collaborators when working with administration, including finance, communications, media, legal, compliance, internal process control, supply chain, continuous improvement experts, and medical directors for quality, patient safety, patient experience, and other areas.

GETTING STARTED

The first step in collaborating with hospital and health system administration is to understand unique pressures and demands, local decision-making processes, and C-suite terminology. If you are new to the organization, consider asking open-ended questions about past performance and history of change, present vision and current processes, as well as future challenges and opportunities.[3] It is also helpful to be well prepared for questions you will receive, such as the regulatory requirements related to your request.

Pressures and Demands

Hospital administrators face numerous financial, reputational, and regulatory pressures. To make a case for antimicrobial stewardship, leaders of the ASP should understand how the program fits into these pressures. For many administrators, financial pressures may be most pressing, so explaining return on investment for an ASP technological or staff investment is vital. Health care faces many challenges related to shifts in outpatient services, patient acuity, and patient payer mix; physician supply and compensation; competition for patients and managed care contracts; and servicing aging equipment, leading to a constant flux of expenses, within which ASP is only a piece. Hospital administrators are also focused on reputation and national ranking provided by such organizations as the US News and the Leapfrog Group, which are influenced by metrics, including mortalities and patient safety scores. The Leapfrog Group now scores hospitals on their commitment to antibiotic stewardship. Some rankings can be affected by health care–associated infections (HAIs) and the hospital epidemiology and infection prevention team are frequently in touch with hospital administration regarding HAI metrics that affect these scores. *Clostridioides difficile* infection (CDI) is a publicly reported metric and a well-developed ASP can help prevent this HAI.[4] Prevention of CDI is an opportunity to work with the infection prevention team and make a case to the administration for the importance of a strong ASP.[5] In addition, meeting regulatory and accreditation requirements is vital to keeping the doors open, and with The Joint Commission's antimicrobial stewardship standard in place since 2017, most health care administrators have increased familiarity with stewardship in this post-accreditation era.[6]

Decision-Making Processes

Before addressing a stewardship-related issue or request with hospital and health system administration, ask strategic questions to understand how the administrative process works. For example, who has formal and informal decision-making rights within the organization? Who are the key opinion leaders in the organization? Are there different approaches for administrative and clinical decisions? What is the usual time line for resource decisions? What is the usual time line for high-level goal-setting decisions? Are decisions typically made in the board room or based on 1-on-1 conversations outside of the boardroom? Frequently, important decisions involve both types of settings. Each hospital or health system has a unique structure and decision-making culture. As much as possible, work within the bounds of the organization's standard structure and culture to be successful.

Resource limitations significantly affect the decision-making process at most hospitals and health systems. Typically, funding antimicrobial stewardship results in not funding another program, initiative, or other personnel,[7] which adds pressure to the antimicrobial stewardship team to show their impact on key metrics, such as length of stay, patient morbidity, and cost. In addition, if it is clear which positions were not funded in favor of ASP funding, strategize ways to assist with the increased burden caused by the unfunded position. For example, if a decision was made to hire an antimicrobial stewardship pharmacist rather than a medicine floor pharmacist, determine ways the antimicrobial stewardship pharmacist can assist with or reduce the medicine floor's workload.

Terminology

It is critical to learn and comprehend common terminology of hospital administration for successful engagement and communication. Partnering with someone in administration or the finance department to better understand these terms and their importance in the organization can be valuable. A few key terms are defined with examples in **Table 1**.

Regulatory Requirements

In 2013, Accreditation Canada expanded the list of Required Organizational Practices to include development and implementation of a program to optimize antimicrobial use and provide good stewardship.[8] In the United States, the Centers for Medicare & Medicaid Services (CMS) required long-term care facilities to develop an infection prevention and control program that includes an antibiotic stewardship program by the end of November 2016.[9] In addition, The Joint Commission implemented a new medication management standard for antibiotic stewardship in 2017 requiring active antibiotic stewardship programs at all accredited hospitals.[10] Critical access hospitals will need to be compliant with the Centers for Disease Control and Prevention (CDC) Core Elements by 2021 to receive flexibility grant funding from the Federal Office of Rural Health Policy via the Medicare Beneficiary Quality Improvement Project (MBQIP).[11,12] In addition, the CMS has approved a new proposal to require hospitals to have ASPs as a condition of participation.

In addition to national standards and accrediting bodies, many organizations publish metrics related to infectious diseases. There are a variety of places to find these metrics, including the Agency for Healthcare Research and Quality (AHRQ), American Medical Association Physician Consortium for Performance Improvement (AMA-PCPI), the CDC, the CMS, Health Resources and Services Administration (HRSA), National Committee for Quality Assurance, The Joint Commission, and the Leapfrog Group. These metrics have been summarized previously.[13] In addition, some states, such as California, Missouri, and Tennessee, have regulatory requirements regarding antimicrobial stewardship. Also, for facilities that are a part of a health system or hospital network, consider the recommendations of governing bodies or task forces for these organizations when determining required elements. For example, the Veterans Health Administration now requires reporting of antimicrobial use data to the National

Table 1
Administrative and financial terminology

Term	Definition
Fiscal year	Instead of a calendar year, companies may use a fiscal year for tax purposes: 12 consecutive months ending on the last day of any month except December. For example, the US federal government fiscal year ends on September 30
Capital expenditure	Those funds disbursed for facilities, equipment, or another physical asset, particularly those related to the delivery of health care. Given the high expense, the cost of these expenditures is often spread over multiple years
Fixed cost[38]	An expense or cost that does not change with an increase or decrease in the number of goods or services produced or sold (eg, salaried employees, hardware, software)
Variable cost[38]	An expense or cost that changes in proportion to production output (eg, medications, medical supplies, sharps disposal containers)
Semivariable cost[38]	An expense or cost that is a mixture of fixed and variable costs. Even if no production occurs, a fixed cost is often still incurred (eg, rapid diagnostic tests, overtime pay)
ROI[39,40]	Reported as a percentage, it is a performance measure to evaluate the efficiency of an investment. The formula is: (Current value of investment − Cost of investment)/Cost of investment
DRG[41]	Classification system for hospital discharges to adjust payments based on appropriate weighting factors. Payment is determined by a hospital's payment rate per case multiplied by the weight of the DRG. Each DRG weight represents the average resources required to care for cases in that DRG compared with all DRGs, and these are adjusted at least annually. The most common coding system is MS-DRG
Case mix index[14]	The sum of the total cost weights of all inpatients per a defined time period divided by the number of admissions. The cost weight of a DRG is defined by dividing the average cost per case of DRG by the mean cost per case on a nationwide level
Value-based purchasing[42]	A CMS payment system that rewards acute care hospitals with incentive payments for quality of care. It is paid for by reducing MS-DRG payments by 2% and distributing this money based on total performance scores. The quality domains are updated each year
HAC reduction program[42]	A Medicare pay-for-performance program in which hospitals are ranked on the following measures: • CMS Recalibrated Patient Safety Indicator • CLABSI • CAUTI • SSI: colon and hysterectomy • MRSA bacteremia • CDI Hospitals with a total HAC score greater than the 75th percentile (ie, the worst-performing quartile) are subject to a 1% payment reduction, applicable to all Medicare discharges (eg, fiscal year 2019 is October 1, 2018, to September 30, 2019)
Stewardship[43]	Stewardship may be used any time a limited resource needs to be used, thus it may be used to signal cost reductions, because money is a limited resource. Consider emphasizing the distinctive nature of antimicrobial stewardship to have a societal impact on antimicrobial resistance that other types of stewardship do not have

(continued on next page)

Table 1 (continued)	
Term	Definition
SWOT analysis[30]	Originally developed based on the results from a Stanford study on Fortune 500 companies to help clarify projects and maximize opportunities

Abbreviations: CAUTI, catheter-associated urinary tract infection; CLABSI, central line-associated bloodstream infection; CMS, Centers for Medicare & Medicaid Services; DRG, diagnosis-related group; HAC, hospital-acquired condition; MRSA, methicillin-resistant *Staphylococcus aureus*; MS-DRG, Medicare Severity DRG; ROI, return on investment; SSI, surgical site infection; SWOT, strengths, weaknesses, opportunities, and threats.

Healthcare Safety Network's Antimicrobial Use Option if the hospital has greater than 30 beds.[14]

PITCHING RESOURCE REQUESTS

In a recent United States survey of 244 antimicrobial stewardship program respondents from 43 states, 151 (62%) somewhat or strongly disagreed with the statement, "The financial resources for my program are adequate."[15] Administrative approval is necessary to obtain these resources. The first step is to get noticed and recognized by key decision makers, which can be achieved by networking with key contacts within the organization or directly setting up a meeting with the hospital administrator, perhaps starting with the chief medical officer. When working on an initial so-called elevator speech, one productive approach is to start with the conclusion and then work backward, or to start with a compelling patient story.[16] Determine the combination of argument types that will best convince the audience. Examples of different types include logos (data and reasoning), ethos (principles, policies, and other rules), and pathos (emotions and meaning).[3] Ask questions about current understanding of antimicrobial stewardship as well, because many administrators may already be familiar with antimicrobial stewardship conceptually but may not have worked at a facility with a formal program.[17] In order to establish productive relationships, multiple interactions are often required. Establish relationships for the long term.

After initial meetings regarding antimicrobial stewardship needs, the next steps are likely to be a formal request made to administration for resources and a business plan developed. A recent publication helps to frame the formal pitch in more detail.[7] A few other published resources and examples are available.[18–20] Sample business plans are available from the Association of Medical Microbiology and Infectious Diseases (AMMI) Canadian Working Group[21] and the Society of Healthcare Epidemiology of America Web site. However, it is also important to review local business plans to better understand the standard form and structure for the institution. Key components of any business plan include executive summary, alignment with mission, vision and values, the business need or rationale (and why the current process is inadequate), program objectives, and details of the financial request.

When considering program objectives, think big and think easy: what are the wide-sweeping problems that have broad impact and what "low-hanging fruit" are easy to change and measurable? Examples might include focusing on specific antimicrobials (high-cost medications), specific antimicrobial combinations (double anaerobic coverage), or common disease states (community-acquired pneumonia).[22] When pitching the needs of antimicrobial stewardship, emphasize the goals of the program as relating to quality, safety, and meeting regulatory requirements. Whenever possible, align goals with issues that are viewed by administration as important or so-called burning-platform issues. Apply innovation to the request: think about so-called outside-the-box opportunities.[23] Avoid business plans that focus solely on eliminating medication costs.[24] Other end points that may be important to administrators include reducing variability in care, shortening length of stay, or providing ongoing education to providers, especially if there are on-site residency training programs. To align with these administration priorities, it is important to communicate with decision makers and key opinion leaders in advance. This preparatory work can also help mitigate the risk of stepping on other key leaders' toes by identifying and involving important collaborators from the beginning. In addition, engagement with external professional societies will also provide insight into national trends and upcoming policy decisions that can assist with the pitch.

For the business plan's financial details, have both a short-term (1 year) and long-term perspective (3–5 years) and describe the potential return on investment (ROI). Examples of ROIs related to infection prevention in the literature are provided in **Table 2**. Consider a phased implementation, especially when enacting change on a health system level.[25] It can be helpful to provide multiple solutions with varying price tags to address the problem, which helps to emphasize the actions and outcomes tied with the financial request and provides options for administrators.

A common barrier to antimicrobial stewardship is lack of financial support for antimicrobial stewardship personnel and other resources.[26] **Table 3** highlights 4 common examples of barriers and some approaches to address these challenges. Regardless of the hurdles, it is important to foster an ongoing relationship with administration and to provide follow-up regarding progress toward goals as well as impediments. If barriers exist, additional discussion and business cases (eg, for new personnel or technology) might be necessary.

Table 2
Examples of returns on investment from infection prevention

Intervention	Health Care–Associated Infection	Reported ROI
Educational modules	CLABSI, SSI, VAP, CAUTI	For every $1 spent on training, the ROI was $236 as cost of avoidance of HAIs[44]
Building single-bed rooms in intensive care unit	HA-MRSA	$418,269 in spending would be avoided through infection reduction in this ICU if all patients hosted in bay rooms were admitted to single-bed rooms[45]
Involvement in a national surgical quality improvement program	SSI	In cumulative savings from averted SSI cases, generating a return of $2.28 (US$3.02) per dollar invested (95% CI, −0.67–7.37)[39]
Public health funding given focused on reducing CLABSI	CLABSI	ROI $1.10–$11.20 per $1 invested[46]

Abbreviations: CI, confidence interval; HA-MRSA, health care–acquired MRSA infection; ICU, intensive care unit; VAP, ventilator-associated pneumonia.

Table 3
Barriers and challenges when asking for resources from administration

Barrier and/or Challenge	Potential Approach
Administration wants to use existing personnel to develop a new antimicrobial stewardship program	Rebuttal: literature supports that infectious diseases–trained personnel achieve greater reductions in antimicrobial use and greater adherence to recommended antimicrobial therapy practices.[47,48] Emphasize the knowledge and skills required of antimicrobial stewardship leaders[49] Compromise: ask for financial support for additional antimicrobial training and/or certification
Administration wants existing dedicated antimicrobials stewardship personnel to expand current responsibilities	Rebuttal: time-in-motion studies or other data support that the current work of the antimicrobial stewardship team is at capacity and there is no bandwidth to expand services Compromise: reduce nonstewardship responsibilities for antimicrobial stewardship leaders, such as clinical weeks of consultation service or providing administrative support. Reassess current projects[50] and determine where some responsibilities can be transitioned to other hospital personnel[51]
Administration is reevaluating current resources for antimicrobial stewardship in a recessive environment	Rebuttal: when antimicrobial stewardship resources are removed, previous gains in control of antimicrobial expenses are lost[52] Compromise: reassess current projects[50] and determine where some responsibilities can be transitioned to other hospital personnel[51]
Administration is resistant to funding new technology to support antimicrobial stewardship	Rebuttal: the purchase of this application would prevent the need to hire additional personnel to accomplish the same objectives. This application would improve patient safety. Other key stakeholders may benefit from using the technology as well, such as infection prevention, pharmacy services, or research groups Compromise: determine whether there are internal informatics resources to develop the reports necessary to accomplish the goal or to adapt current applications for antimicrobial stewardship use[53]

DEFINING STRUCTURE, PERSONNEL TASKS, AND JOB DESCRIPTIONS

It is important for hospital and health system administration to understand and appreciate the institutional value provided by the antimicrobial stewardship team and the resources needed for the team to be successful. For this to occur, consider personnel tasks and job descriptions, material needs and budgets, and the reporting structure of the antimicrobial stewardship program. The multidisciplinary nature of the ASP team is a key element that makes stewardship programs impactful and complex, and investment in protecting time of the leaders of the ASP is associated with success.[2,6] The CDC's Core Elements of Hospital Antibiotic Stewardship Programs recommend the appointment of a stewardship program leader (typically a physician) responsible for program outcomes and a single pharmacy leader to co-lead the program.[27] Formal training in infectious diseases and/or antimicrobial stewardship is beneficial but not required. Providing financial support for these positions is a component of leadership commitment and administrative support.[2] Although there is no specific guidance on the recommended full-time equivalents (FTEs) for these positions, a summary of recent literature regarding personnel resources is provided in **Table 4**.

Often, the expected day-to-day tasks of an ASP help determine the likelihood of obtaining proposed resources. Therefore, it is important to consider the specific responsibilities of antimicrobial stewardship personnel early in the development or expansion of a program. These expectations should be compiled into clear job descriptions. Sample job descriptions and postings can be found through professional organization Web sites, such as the Society for Healthcare Epidemiology of America and the Society of Infectious Diseases Pharmacists, and networking with fellow ASP colleagues, although descriptions need to be modified to fit the needs and cultures of specific organizations. Clearly communicating essential day-to-day functions and proactively sharing patient safety stories via a written quarterly update, presentations at a quarterly meeting, or routinely scheduled brief 1-on-1 meetings with quality, medical, and pharmacy leadership are successful strategies to reemphasize core personnel and the impact of their day-to-day responsibilities. This proactive strategy may improve chances of obtaining resources and avoids only interacting with administration when resources are needed.

Information Technology and Data Management Support

In addition to standard personnel, most ASPs require additional resources to accomplish their day-to-day work, as well as their quality improvement initiatives. Day-to-day work can be supported by internal access to data and reports and augmented by add-on or integrated computer decision-support systems. Use of the electronic health record for alerts and data tracking requires prioritization of internal information technology resources. In addition, data analysis and data management expertise are additional resources necessary to show impact on a larger scale with broader initiatives. When defining structure, it is important to keep in mind not only the physician and pharmacist personnel resources that are needed but these additional resources as well.

Reporting Structure

Where antimicrobial stewardship fits within a hospital or health system varies based on the organization. Helpful questions for antimicrobial stewardship leaders to consider when determining where stewardship fits include whether reporting relationships help align effort; whether it is clear who is accountable for what; and whether the kinds of achievements that matter most are being measured and rewarded (are there the right incentives?).[3] Ideally, the reporting structure would include access to key decision makers as well as visibility and support from a multidisciplinary audience, which may need to be accomplished through more than 1 reporting avenue. For example, the medical director of antimicrobial stewardship may report to the chief medical officer or the chief quality officer and the lead antimicrobial stewardship pharmacist may report to the chief pharmacy officer; however, the 2 co-leads may also report together to the pharmacy and therapeutics committee, the infection control committee, the medication safety committee, the quality board, and other aligned groups. Because the infection prevention team has an established reporting structure either directly within the quality department or within the division of infectious diseases, it can be used as a model. One study reported that most infection prevention departments report within the department of medicine, but some also report to quality

Table 4
Antimicrobial stewardship staffing ratios

Reference	Country	Methodology	Recommendation
Ten Oever et al,[26] 2018	The Netherlands	Semistructured interviews, an electronic survey, and face-to-face consensus meeting focusing on antimicrobial stewardship tasks and associated time requirements	Start-up investment: 100–135 h Maintenance (1 stewardship objective): • 300-bed hospital: 0.87–1.11 combined FTE • 750-bed hospital: 1.15–1.39 combined FTE • 1200-bed hospital: 1.43–1.68 combined FTE Maintenance (3 stewardship objectives): • 300-bed hospital: 1.25–1.49 combined FTE • 750-bed hospital: 2.09–2.33 combined FTE • 1200-bed hospital: 2.93–3.18 combined FTE
Doernberg et al,[15] 2018	United States	Cross-sectional survey and association between FTE and antimicrobial stewardship program results	Each 0.5 increase in combined FTE availability results in a 1.48-fold increase in the odds of showing effectiveness (95% CI, 1.06–2.07) Proposed minimum FTEs for antimicrobial stewardship: • 100-bed to 300-bed hospital: 1.4 combined FTE • 301-bed to 500-bed hospital: 1.6 combined FTE • 501-bed to 1000-bed hospital: 2.6 combined FTE • >1000-bed hospital: 4.0 combined FTE
Wong et al,[54] 2018	Canada	Survey of 15 pediatric hospitals and assessment of current FTE allotment	Hospitals ranged from 38 to 484 beds and designated combined FTE ranged from 0.0 to 1.8 (median, 0.7 FTE)
Morris et al,[21] 2018	Canada	Narrative review of the literature and expert working group consensus decision-making process	Recommended FTEs per 1000 acute care beds: • Physicians: 1.0 FTE • Pharmacists: 3.0 FTE • Administrative support: 0.5 FTE • Data analysts: 0.4 FTE
Echevarria et al,[55] 2017	United States	Time-in-motion studies for common activities at 12 validation sites and expert opinion for others	Pharmacists: median 1.1 FTE per 100 occupied beds (interquartile range, 1.0–1.47), of which approximately 70% was related to patient care and 30% to program management Note: task force recommends 0.25 physician FTE per 100 occupied beds

(continued on next page)

Table 4 (*continued*)			
Reference	Country	Methodology	Recommendation
Le Coz et al,[56] 2016	France	Cross-sectional nationwide survey of 65 hospitals to define optimal standards	Recommended 6.7 FTE per 1000 acute care beds: • ID specialists: 3.6 FTE per 1000 acute care beds • Pharmacists: 2.5 FTE per 1000 beds • Microbiologists: 0.6 FTE per 1000 beds

Abbreviation: ID, infectious diseases.

management or nursing.[28] It is the opinion of the authors that structuring antimicrobial stewardship within the quality department is ideal, given the aim to improve the quality and safety of care for patients who receive antibiotics and/or are managed for infections.

In addition to reporting to leadership, bidirectional communication is often effective and can be achieved by inviting hospital administration to the antimicrobial stewardship committee. One health system promotes the inclusion of the chief executive officer as an ad hoc member of the antimicrobial stewardship program, and chief medical officers are members of the team in half of its facilities.[25]

ONGOING ACTIONS AND COMMUNICATION

Once resources have been approved and a structure established, the antimicrobial stewardship team needs to deliver results. To do this successfully, the antimicrobial stewardship leaders need to hone the skills of goal setting, follow-through, and communication.

Goal Setting

New ASPs should start with initial goals that are feasible and represent low-hanging fruit. When prioritizing potential goals, a good place to start are those that assist with meeting regulatory requirements. Other factors that affect the likelihood of success should also be considered, including the narrowness of scope, estimated time and resources needed, data availability, resource availability, number of areas involved, and complexity of the project.[29] Established programs have more freedom for innovation and need to be strategic about how to take on new goals while maintaining, modifying, or retiring other responsibilities. All programs benefit from a thoughtful and strategic approach to goal setting. Alignment with organizational priorities is recommended. Thinking innovatively with an expanded scope is encouraged, such as goals that involve vaccination, methods of microbiologic sampling, value-based purchasing, and discharge counseling. If a goal involves multiple disciplines or collaboration, start early in pitching potential goals to stakeholders because departments may plan their goals 6 months or more in advance.

According to the John Whitmore model for goal setting, in addition to the traditional SMART (specific, measurable, attainable, realistic, and time phased) criteria, also consider making goals PURE (positively stated, understood, relevant, ethical) and CLEAR (challenging, legal, environmentally sound, agreed, and recorded).[30] In antimicrobial stewardship, one of the biggest challenges in creating a SMART goal is making it measurable. Two approaches can be used: leveraging already collected metrics and developing new simplified metrics. An example of a metric that is already collected for public reporting is *C difficile* infections. An example of a simplified metric is an electronically pulled raw assessment of acute kidney injury in patients receiving vancomycin, which can be trended over time and takes fewer resources than a metric that takes into account all potential confounders.[31] Another challenge is making a goal realistic: avoid primary metrics that might be beyond the influence and control of the ASP, such as reducing antimicrobial resistance rates.

It may be helpful to think about goals in terms of a primary "big-picture" mission statement and the smaller objectives and steps necessary to achieve this goal. These smaller objectives and steps can be portrayed in shorter-term aims that are often related to process measures (**Table 5** for examples). Process measures are measures of whether an activity has been accomplished, such as acknowledgment of an alert or use of a decision-support tool.[32] For larger projects or initiatives, some institutions may require that specific templates be used to help break projects down into smaller aims and processes as well as communication with leadership (eg, A3 strategy form, a tool in lean process improvement). It is recommended to use templates familiar to the organization.

Follow-Through

Once goals are set, the work of follow-through begins. In developing an implementation plan, recommendations from implementation science can be helpful. Implementation science is defined as the scientific study of methods to promote the systematic uptake of research findings and other evidence-based practice into routine practice.[33] Two ways to incorporate implementation science into daily stewardship activity are to use implementation strategies and outcomes. There are more than 73 implementation strategies to choose from; however, some of the most common ones used in antimicrobial stewardship are audit and provision of feedback, conduct ongoing training, create new clinical teams, develop educational materials, distribute educational materials, and remind clinicians about stewardship-related issues.[34] Outcomes to measure the success of implementation include acceptability, appropriateness, adoption, cost, feasibility, fidelity, penetration, and sustainability.[35] Examples of how these outcomes

Table 5
Example mission and aim statements

General Mission Statement	Aim Statement
Increase the timely and appropriate transition of highly bioavailable antimicrobials from the intravenous to the oral route, while also optimizing the alert burden for frontline pharmacists	To increase the percentage of oral days of levofloxacin from 30% to 50% in the next 6 mo by improving the average pharmacist positive action response time to intravenous to oral alert triggers to <4 h
Support our organization's mission by improving care for patients who are admitted with a diagnosis of sepsis by reducing 30-d all-cause readmissions	Decrease the volume of 30-d readmissions for medical-surgical patients admitted with a primary diagnosis of sepsis by 5% by focusing on 3 focused improvements in the discharge process
Optimize appropriate clindamycin use for surgical prophylaxis in orthopedic patients	Increase appropriate clindamycin use to 85% in the next 6 mo by improving the percentage of patients who have a complete allergy history taken from 25% to 75%

can be measured include surveys, interviews, and tracking usage data. These metrics are helpful in determining uptake and effectiveness of the intervention and adjusting iteratively when change is not realized. Scheduled, routine tracking of progress on deliverables helps to redirect the intervention if a corrective action plan is needed.

Accountability for outcomes by the antimicrobial stewardship leader is commonly based on influence rather than authority. The 3 keys to influence are (1) focusing on and measuring the right thing, (2) defining vital behaviors, and (3) engaging all 6 sources of influence.[36] The 6 sources of influence center on motivation and ability on personal, social, and structural levels. Strategies such as creating clear and compelling goals, telling moving stories, assisting others with deliberate practice, providing encouragement, as well as creating a structure to make it easy to do the right thing are effective examples of leveraging influence and improving accountability relevant to antimicrobial stewardship.

Communication

Ideally, frequent updates and feedback are integrated into current reporting structures. When significant barriers are confronted (eg, difficult prescribers, technologic hurdles, or resource limitations) it is important to seek assistance from administration. Routine communication helps to promote antimicrobial stewardship equally during both smooth and struggling phases, which can improve relationships with administration. These updates are best if concise with a clear message.[7] In addition, a written annual report to administration is recommended.[37] An annual report, with executive summary and supporting details, is beneficial both as a communication tool as well as documentation for future reference.

SUMMARY

The first step in collaborating with hospital and health system administration is to understand their structure and speak their language. Pitching resource requests requires major interactions with administration, so being prepared to present clearly and concisely and address key questions is important for success. When determining the pitch, consider resources for information technology support in addition to personnel requests. Thoughtfully consider the best reporting structure for the ASP, which should include a defined relationship with the organization's quality department. In addition, develop an ongoing relationship with administrators to highlight successes and to gain their assistance in addressing challenges.

DISCLOSURES

The authors report no relevant disclosures.

REFERENCES

1. Goff DA, Karam GH, Haines ST. Impact of a national antimicrobial stewardship mentoring program: insights and lessons learned. Am J Health Syst Pharm 2017;74:224–31.
2. Pollack LA, van Santen KL, Weiner LM, et al. Antibiotic Stewardship Programs in U.S. acute care hospitals: findings from the 2014 National Healthcare Safety Network Annual Hospital Survey. Clin Infect Dis 2016;63:443–9.
3. Michael DW. The first 90 days. Boston: Harvard Business Review Press; 2013.
4. Baur D, Gladstone BP, Burkert F, et al. Effect of antibiotic stewardship on the incidence of infection and colonisation with antibiotic-resistant bacteria and

Clostridium difficile infection: a systematic review and meta-analysis. Lancet Infect Dis 2017;17:990–1001.

5. Louh IK, Greendyke WG, Hermann EA, et al. Clostridium Difficile infection in acute care hospitals: systematic review and best practices for prevention. Infect Control Hosp Epidemiol 2017;38:476–82.

6. Goff DA, Kullar R, Bauer KA, et al. Eight habits of highly effective antimicrobial stewardship programs to meet the joint commission standards for hospitals. Clin Infect Dis 2017;64:1134–9.

7. Spellberg B, Bartlett JG, Gilbert DN. How to pitch an antibiotic stewardship program to the hospital c-suite. Open Forum Infect Dis 2016;3:ofw210.

8. Canada A. Required Organizational Practices (ROP) handbook 2017 – Version 2. Available at: https://accreditation.ca/required-organizational-practices/. Accessed March 4, 2019.

9. Centers for Medicare and Medicaid Services. Medicare and medicaid programs reform of requirements for longterm care facilities, vol. 81. Department of Health and Human Services, CMS; 2016. FR 68688.

10. The Joint Commission. Approved: new antimicrobial stewardship standard. Joint Commission Perspectives; 2016. Available at: https://www.jointcommission.org/assets/1/6/New_Antimicrobial_Stewardship_Standard.pdf. Accessed February 1, 2018.

11. Centers for Medicare and Medicaid Services. Medicare and Medicaid Programs; Hospital and Critical Access Hospital (CAH) changes to promote innovation, flexibility, and improvement in patient care. 2016. Available at: https://www.federalregister.gov/documents/2016/06/16/2016-13925/medicare-and-medicaid-programs-hospital-and-critical-access-hospital-cah-changes-to-promote. Accessed February 1, 2018.

12. National Rural Health Resource Center. MBQIP new required measure FY2018-2021. 2017. Available at: https://www.ruralcenter.org/file/antibiotics-stewardship-measures-mbqip-fiscal-years-2018-2021. Accessed February 1, 2018.

13. Nagel JL, Stevenson JG, Eiland EH 3rd, et al. Demonstrating the value of antimicrobial stewardship programs to hospital administrators. Clin Infect Dis 2014;59(Suppl 3):S146–53.

14. Kuster SP, Ruef C, Bollinger AK, et al. Correlation between case mix index and antibiotic use in hospitals. J Antimicrob Chemother 2008;62:837–42.

15. Doernberg SB, Abbo LM, Burdette SD, et al. Essential resources and strategies for antibiotic stewardship programs in the acute care setting. Clin Infect Dis 2018;67:1168–74.

16. Rieger E, Aggarwal P, Cameron C. Scientific elevator speeches: a communication and critical thinking tool. Med Educ 2017;51:559.

17. Buckel WR, Hersh AL, Pavia AT, et al. Antimicrobial stewardship knowledge, attitudes, and practices among health care professionals at small community hospitals. Hosp Pharm 2016;51:149–57.

18. McQuillen DP, Petrak RM, Wasserman RB, et al. The value of infectious diseases specialists: non–patient care activities. Clin Infect Dis 2008;47:1051–63.

19. Scheetz MH, Bolon MK, Postelnick M, et al. Cost-effectiveness analysis of an antimicrobial stewardship team on bloodstream infections: a probabilistic analysis. J Antimicrob Chemother 2009;63:816–25.

20. Dellit TH, Owens RC, McGowan JE Jr, et al. Infectious Diseases Society of America and the Society for Healthcare Epidemiology of America guidelines for

developing an institutional program to enhance antimicrobial stewardship. Clin Infect Dis 2007;44:159–77.

21. Morris AM, Rennert-May E, Dalton B, et al. Rationale and development of a business case for antimicrobial stewardship programs in acute care hospital settings. Antimicrob Resist Infect Control 2018;7:104.

22. Patel PK. Applying the horizontal and vertical paradigm to antimicrobial stewardship. Infect Control Hosp Epidemiol 2017;38:532–3.

23. Hamilton KW, Fishman NO. Antimicrobial stewardship interventions: thinking inside and outside the box. Infect Dis Clin North Am 2014;28:301–13.

24. Pulcini C, Morel CM, Tacconelli E, et al. Human resources estimates and funding for antibiotic stewardship teams are urgently needed. Clin Microbiol Infect 2017; 23:785–7.

25. Burgess LH, Miller K, Cooper M, et al. Phased implementation of an antimicrobial stewardship program for a large community hospital system. Am J Infect Control 2019;47:69–73.

26. Ten Oever J, Harmsen M, Schouten J, et al. Human resources required for antimicrobial stewardship teams: a Dutch consensus report. Clin Microbiol Infect 2018;24:1273–9.

27. Centers for Disease Control and Prevention. Core elements of hospital antibiotic stewardship programs. 2014. Available at: http://www.cdc.gov/getsmart/healthcare/implementation/core-elements.html. Accessed February 1, 2019.

28. Stone PW, Dick A, Pogorzelska M, et al. Staffing and structure of infection prevention and control programs. Am J Infect Control 2009;37:351–7.

29. Scholtes J, Joiner B, Streibel B. The team handbook. 3rd edition. Edison (NJ): Oriel STAT A MATRIX; 2010.

30. Krogerus M, Tschappeler R. The decision book. New York: W. W. Norton & Company; 2012.

31. Heil EL, Claeys KC, Mynatt RP, et al. Making the change to area under the curve-based vancomycin dosing. Am J Health Syst Pharm 2018;75:1986–95.

32. Langley G, Moen R, Nolan K, et al. The improvement guide. 2nd edition. San Francisco (CA): Jossey-Bass; 2009.

33. Eccles MP, Foy R, Sales A, et al. Implementation science six years on–our evolving scope and common reasons for rejection without review. Implement Sci 2012;7:71.

34. Powell BJ, Waltz TJ, Chinman MJ, et al. A refined compilation of implementation strategies: results from the Expert Recommendations for Implementing Change (ERIC) project. Implement Sci 2015;10:21.

35. Proctor E, Silmere H, Raghavan R, et al. Outcomes for implementation research: conceptual distinctions, measurement challenges, and research agenda. Adm Policy Ment Health 2011;38:65–76.

36. Grenny J, Patterson K, Maxfield D, et al. Influencer: the new science of leading change. 2nd edition. San Francisco (CA): McGraw-Hill; 2013. Paperback.

37. Pollack LA, Plachouras D, Sinkowitz-Cochran R, et al. A concise set of structure and process indicators to assess and compare antimicrobial stewardship programs among EU and US hospitals: results from a multinational expert panel. Infect Control Hosp Epidemiol 2016;37:1201–11.

38. Ryan P, Skally M, Duffy F, et al. Evaluation of fixed and variable hospital costs due to Clostridium difficile infection: institutional incentives and directions for future research. J Hosp Infect 2017;95:415–20.

39. van Katwyk S, Thavorn K, Coyle D, et al. The return of investment of hospital-based surgical quality improvement programs in reducing surgical site infection

at a Canadian tertiary-care hospital. Infect Control Hosp Epidemiol 2019;40: 125–32.

40. Dik JW, Hendrix R, Friedrich AW, et al. Cost-minimization model of a multidisciplinary antibiotic stewardship team based on a successful implementation on a urology ward of an academic hospital. PLoS One 2015;10:e0126106.

41. Hebbinckuys E, Marissal JP, Preda C, et al. Assessing the burden of Clostridium difficile infections for hospitals. J Hosp Infect 2018;98:29–35.

42. Hsu HE, Wang R, Jentzsch MS, et al. Association between value-based incentive programs and catheter-associated urinary tract infection rates in the critical care setting. JAMA 2019;321:509–11.

43. Dyar OJ, Moran-Gilad J, Greub G, et al. Diagnostic stewardship: are we using the right term? Clin Microbiol Infect 2019;25:272–3.

44. Sundaram KR, Nair P, Kumar RK, et al. Improving outcomes and reducing costs by modular training in infection control in a resource-limited setting. Int J Qual Health Care 2012;24:641–8.

45. Sadatsafavi H, Niknejad B, Zadeh R, et al. Do cost savings from reductions in nosocomial infections justify additional costs of single-bed rooms in intensive care units? A simulation case study. J Crit Care 2016;31:194–200.

46. Whittington MD, Bradley CJ, Atherly AJ, et al. Value of public health funding in preventing hospital bloodstream infections in the United States. Am J Public Health 2017;107:1764–9.

47. Stenehjem E, Hersh AL, Buckel WR, et al. Impact of implementing antibiotic stewardship programs in 15 small hospitals: a cluster-randomized intervention. Clin Infect Dis 2018;67:525–32.

48. Bessesen MT, Ma A, Clegg D, et al. Antimicrobial stewardship programs: comparison of a program with infectious diseases pharmacist support to a program with a geographic pharmacist staffing model. Hosp Pharm 2015;50:477–83.

49. Cosgrove SE, Hermsen ED, Rybak MJ, et al. Guidance for the knowledge and skills required for antimicrobial stewardship leaders. Infect Control Hosp Epidemiol 2014;35:1444–51.

50. Rose H, Michael DW. Too many projects: why companies won't let bad projects die. Harvard Business Review 2018.

51. DiDiodato G, McAthur L. Transition from a dedicated to a non-dedicated, ward-based pharmacist antimicrobial stewardship programme model in a non-academic hospital and its impact on length of stay of patients admitted with pneumonia: a prospective observational study. BMJ Open Qual 2017;6:e000060.

52. Standiford HC, Chan S, Tripoli M, et al. Antimicrobial stewardship at a large tertiary care academic medical center: cost analysis before, during, and after a 7-year program. Infect Control Hosp Epidemiol 2012;33:338–45.

53. Rawlins MDM, Raby E, Sanfilippo FM, et al. Adaptation of a hospital electronic referral system for antimicrobial stewardship prospective audit and feedback rounds. Int J Qual Health Care 2018;30:637–41.

54. Wong J, Timberlake K, Boodhan S, et al. Canadian pediatric antimicrobial stewardship programs: current resources and implementation characteristics. Infect Control Hosp Epidemiol 2018;39:350–4.

55. Echevarria K, Groppi J, Kelly AA, et al. Development and application of an objective staffing calculator for antimicrobial stewardship programs in the Veterans Health Administration. Am J Health Syst Pharm 2017;74:1785–90.

56. Le Coz P, Carlet J, Roblot F, et al. Human resources needed to perform antimicrobial stewardship teams' activities in French hospitals. Med Mal Infect 2016;46: 200–6.

Bugs and Drugs
Collaboration Between Infection Prevention and Antibiotic Stewardship

Erin M. Gentry, PharmD, BCPS[a],*, Shelley Kester, MHA, BSN, RN, CIC[b],
Kristin Fischer, BM, MM[c], Lisa E. Davidson, MD[d],
Catherine L. Passaretti, MD[e]

KEYWORDS

- Antibiotic stewardship • Infection prevention • Collaboration • MDROs
- Diagnostic stewardship

KEY POINTS

- Collaborative efforts between infection prevention (IP) and antibiotic stewardship (ASP) programs maximize efficiency and impact in the battle to prevent further antimicrobial resistance.
- Antibiotic stewardship and IP programs share common goals and challenges.
- Collaboration between ASP and IP has been fruitful in multidrug-resistant organism reduction, surgical site infection and *Clostridioides difficile* infection preventions, and education on asymptomatic bacteriuria.

Antimicrobial resistance is one of the largest public health threats of modern day with implications extending globally. Although the knowledge that bacteria can quickly develop resistance to antibiotics has been recognized since the 1940s and basic tenets of contemporary infection prevention (IP) programs can be traced back to staphylococcal outbreaks in England in the 1950s, modern-day antibiotic stewardship programs (ASPs) did not exist until the late 1990s. The term antibiotic stewardship was first used in print by 2 hospital epidemiologists, John McGowan and Dale Gerding, in 1996 to highlight the double-edged sword of ever-rising rates of multidrug-resistant organisms (MDROs) and the concomitant decline in antibiotic

[a] Antimicrobial Support Network, Carolinas Medical Center, Department of Pharmacy Services, Atrium Health, 1000 Blythe Boulevard, Charlotte, NC 28203, USA; [b] Infection Prevention, Division of Quality, Atrium Health, 1616 Scott Avenue, Charlotte, NC 28203, USA; [c] Department of Medicine, Division of Infectious Diseases, Atrium Health, 1540 Garden Terrace, Suite 209, Charlotte, NC 28203, USA; [d] Antimicrobial Support Network, Internal Medicine, Division of Infectious Diseases, Atrium Health, 1540 Garden Terrace, Suite 211, Charlotte, NC 28203, USA; [e] Health System Infection Prevention, Internal Medicine, Division of Infectious Diseases, Atrium Health, 1616 Scott Avenue, Charlotte, NC 28203, USA
* Corresponding author.
E-mail address: Erin.Gentry@atriumhealth.org

Infect Dis Clin N Am 34 (2020) 17–30
https://doi.org/10.1016/j.idc.2019.10.001
0891-5520/20/Published by Elsevier Inc.
id.theclinics.com

treatment options.[1] Widespread push for ASP started even later when the Centers for Disease Control and Prevention (CDC) brought national attention to antibiotic resistance with the release of Antibiotic Resistance Threats in the United States, 2013.[2] To combat the urgent threat of resistant organisms, the federal government formed the Presidential Advisory Council on Combating Antibiotic-Resistant Bacteria in 2015 to develop a national action plan, which was then followed with the White House Forum on Antibiotic Stewardship.[3–5]

The growth of ASP has been fast and furious over the past 10 years. However, the optimal structure of ASPs and division of labor with other quality improvement groups, such as IP, patient safety, and performance improvement, remains unclear. In particular, ASP and IP programs are naturally complementary, but few data exist as to the optimal interplay between the 2 areas at either the facility or health system level. For many facilities, ASP and IP essentially function as a unit with shared resources, goals, and reporting structures. In other facilities, there may be a greater separation with different reporting structures, goals, and funding streams. Additional programs fall somewhere in between. With the ever-increasing complexity of health care, identifying and acting on collaborative efforts that maximize efficiency and impact of multidisciplinary stakeholders is essential to successfully combat antimicrobial resistance.

Although there will always be variability in ASP and IP interactions based on facility and resource-specific factors, the goal of this article was to review available guidance on structures and activities of ASP and IP programs, identify any overlap of guidelines, identify shared goals and challenges, describe our approach to this evolving collaboration, and highlight the areas in which the ASP-IP dyad has shown to be successful.

ANTIBIOTIC STEWARDSHIP PROGRAM AND INFECTION PREVENTION PROGRAM STRUCTURE AND GOALS

Available guidance from groups like the Infectious Diseases Society of America (IDSA), the Society for Healthcare Epidemiology of America, and the Association for Professionals in Infection Prevention and Control reflect more similarities than differences in recommended components of ASP and IP programs (**Fig. 1**). Support from hospital administration, accountability, strong leadership of the program by trained physician

Applicability of Core Elements of Hospital Antibiotic Stewardship Programs in Infection Prevention Programs		ASP	IP Program
Leadership Commitment:	Dedicating necessary human, financial and information technology resources	✓	✓
Accountability:	Appointing a single leader responsible for program outcomes. Experience with successful programs shows that a physician leader is effective	✓	✓
Drug Expertise:	Appointing a single pharmacist leader responsible for working to improve antibiotic use	✓	✗
Action:	Implementing at least one recommended action to improve outcomes	✓	✓
Tracking:	Surveillance for process and outcome measures	✓	✓
Reporting:	Regular reporting of data to doctors, nurses, and relevant staff	✓	✓
Education:	Educating clinicians on recommended guidelines	✓	✓

Fig. 1. Applicability of core elements of hospital ASPs in IP programs.

or pharmacist subject matter experts, ability to track and deliver data, and education are key components of both types of programs.[6–14] Infection preventionists spend nearly half of their time performing surveillance and analyzing data on health care–associated infection and multidrug-resistant organisms, 15% of their time on educational activities, and 15% of their time in policy development.[15] ASP pharmacists may have a slightly different focus, but their day-to-day activities are very much similar (Fig. 2).

ASPs and IP programs are often held accountable for shared goals. The Centers for Medicare and Medicaid Services, as well as many states, publicly report hospital performance on certain health care–associated infection outcome measures impacted by both ASP and IP initiatives, and mandate submission of associated data through the CDC National Health Safety Network (NHSN) database. Performance on hospital-onset *Clostridioides difficile* infection (CDI), hospital-onset methicillin-resistant *Staphylococcus aureus* (MRSA) bacteremia, deep and organ space colon and abdominal hysterectomy surgical site infections (SSIs), catheter-associated urinary tract infections (CAUTIs), and central line–associated bloodstream infections into value-based purchasing has prompted enhanced C-suite attention to performance and improvement work on these measures by both ASPs and IP programs.[16,17] Ultimately, the NHSN database will be a common repository for both IP and ASP data tracking and national comparison, further tying together IP and ASP outcome data.[18]

ANTIBIOTIC STEWARDSHIP PROGRAM AND INFECTION PREVENTION PROGRAM OPPORTUNITIES AND SHARED CHALLENGES

The overlap between IP and ASP program structure, activities, and goals provides many opportunities for collaboration. In facilities developing new ASP programs in which IP programs are already well established, ASPs can use those preexisting IP structures to build on.[19–21] Especially with the rise of nontraditional ASP programs with shared responsibility with nursing, infection preventionists, and hospital epidemiologists can help bridge gaps and make connections.[22,23] Resources, such as data

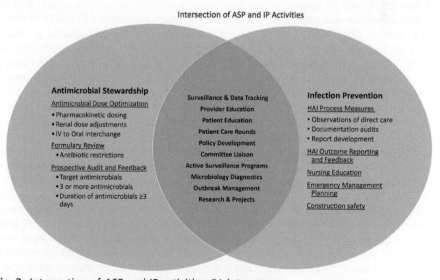

Fig. 2. Intersection of ASP and IP activities. IV, intravenous.

mining software, often can be leveraged by both. Shared educational efforts and protocols between the 2 programs can allow for greater potential impact and reach. Beyond program development, IP surveillance data on MDROs and CDI can be used to monitor and support the impact of both IP and ASP initiatives.[19,20]

Although many areas are ripe for collaboration between IP and ASP, implementation of both types of programs can be extremely challenging. Lack of both funding and dedicated, trained personnel haunts both IP and ASP program development and growth.[24] Literature on optimal staffing ratios for infection preventionists and hospital epidemiologists,[25–27] as well as ASP pharmacists and physicians,[28–30] is limited, and many facilities do not meet those recommended staffing ratios for either type of program. Other shared barriers include limited power to implement change, lack of timely information technology support, opposition from health care workers on initiatives, difficulty in implementing meaningful education, and challenges with communicating recommendations/policies to health care workers.[24,31] Finally, different, and multiple, reporting structures between IP programs and ASPs, as well as between physician leads and infection preventionists/pharmacists, can also be a barrier to collaboration.

OUR APPROACH

Atrium Health is a large health care system that owns 11 acute care hospitals, 2 behavioral health centers, 4 acute rehabilitation facilities, 5 skilled nursing facilities, and more than 400 outpatient clinics. Owned acute care facilities range in size from 15 to more than 800 beds, with services including adult and pediatric bone marrow transplantation, pediatric specialty care, neonatal intensive care units, solid organ transplantation, trauma, and residency programs in multiple areas. Atrium Health creates internal awareness and implements interventions as a system-wide collaborative, including both IP and the system-wide ASP, known as the Antimicrobial Support Network (ASN).

The IP program at Atrium has a centralized structure that consists of an overarching program medical director and assistant vice president who coordinate across facilities within the health system, 2 hospital epidemiologists, 3 directors, 3 data coordinators, 5 IP assistants who all cover multiple facilities in common geographic areas, and 23 infection preventionists dedicated to individual facilities. In addition, IP and ASN share a data analyst who helps with tracking and trending of data and special projects. Except for the medical director and hospital epidemiologists who report through the medical group, the remainder of the IP team reports to the Quality Department. Facility IPs, in addition to reporting through quality, also report to their facility nursing executive and chief medical officers. With multiple lanes of authority comes competing initiatives and request for time. Each individual facility has an IP committee that reports up to the medical executive committee and includes ASN representatives who share data and current initiatives at each meeting.

The Atrium Health ASN began in our facilities in 2013 and in many ways mirrored the structure already in place for the Atrium Health IP program. ASN is also a centralized program organized into 4 divisions to provide services. Like the Atrium Health IP program, ASN has a medical director and 2 physicians who report through the medical group. Under the physician leads, the program consists of a pharmacy program manager who oversees 12 adult and 2 pediatric pharmacists (**Fig. 3**). In contrast to IP, ASN pharmacists report through pharmacy administration at the health system level, and approval for initiatives is routed through the Pharmacy and Therapeutics Committee. ASN pharmacists in this integrated network model function as an independent operational unit, rather than reporting through individual facility pharmacy departments.

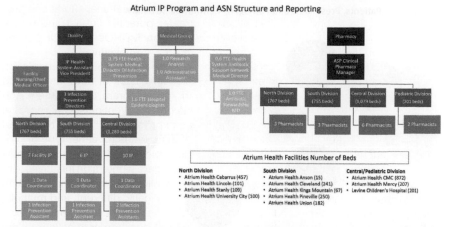

Fig. 3. Atrium IP program and ASN structure and reporting. CMC, Carolinas Medical Center; FTE, full-time equivalent.

ASN provides a combination of prospective audit with intervention and feedback, along with some components of antimicrobial restrictions for the most recent formulary additions. Added responsibilities include interpretation of rapid diagnostic blood culture results with direct communication with microbiology, implementation of an *S aureus* bacteremia bundle, coordination with facility pharmacy divisions and pharmacy quality committees, research, and provision of education programs for clinicians, nurses, and patients in both the acute care and ambulatory care settings.

Given the different reporting structure for IP and ASN in our health system, and, in an effort to better coordinate all facets of infectious disease interventions at our facilities, we have developed a system-wide infectious disease task force called 3P (patients, prescribers, and pathogens). This task force consists of a multidisciplinary team of key stakeholders and is led by the health system chief medical officer and infectious diseases leaders (**Fig. 4**). The goal of 3P is to rapidly assess system infectious disease issues, problem solve, coordinate interventions, implement solutions, and assess response. This multidisciplinary structure has helped acquire high-level key stakeholders at the table and functions to set combined goals, standardize initiatives related to infectious diseases, and ensure progress across the health care system through pharmacy, nursing, quality, and the medical group. Although helpful in a complex health care system, the committee does not have official voting power or budget and as such faces some limitations.

Although the preceding is the approach we have chosen to take, many variations of IP program and ASP interactions exist, and there are some data on how and where those interactions can be effective. There are several healthcare-associated infection outcomes whereby collaboration between IP and ASP has been shown to be productive. Those areas include MDRO prevention, SSI prevention initiatives, diagnostic stewardship initiatives related to CDI, and educational initiatives related to asymptomatic bacteriuria (**Fig. 5**).

MULTIDRUG-RESISTANT ORGANISM PREVENTION

The spread of MDROs is one of the biggest public health challenges facing health care today, and overuse of broad-spectrum antibiotics, contaminated pieces of equipment, and poor adherence to IP protocols have all been suggested as

Patients, Prescribers and Pathogens Committee Structure

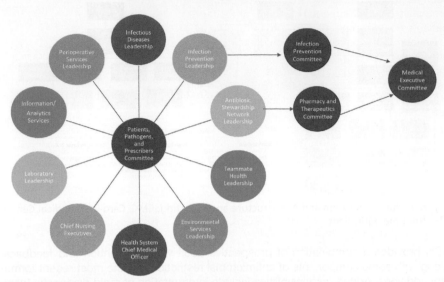

Fig. 4. Patients, prescribers, and pathogens committee structure.

contributors in both endemic and outbreak settings.[32,33] Carbapenem-resistant Enterobacteriaceae (CRE), extended spectrum beta lactamase-producing (ESBL) Enterobacteriaceae, and Vancomycin-resistant *Enterococcus* have been flagged by the CDC and World Health Organization as critical or urgent threats.[2] Limiting the development of these organisms requires preemptive action in the form of antibiotic stewardship and effective coordinated response once organisms or outbreaks are identified in the form of IP. As part of a multipronged effort to control CRE, CDC

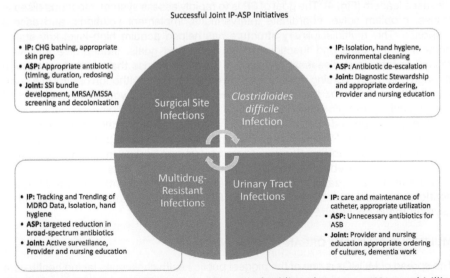

Fig. 5. Successful joint IP-ASP initiatives. CHG, chlorhexidine gluconate; MSSA, methicillin-sensitive *Staphylococcus aureus*.

guidance includes both control of broad-spectrum antibiotics and IP interventions, such as rigorous hand hygiene, strict contact isolation, active surveillance, increased emphasis on environmental cleaning, and cohorting of health care workers caring for patients colonized or infected with CRE.[34,35]

Beyond CRE control, several studies have shown that implementation of ASPs can effectively reduce incidence of organisms such as MRSA, imipenem-resistant *Pseudomonas*, ESBL-producing organisms, and CDI.[36,37] Fluoroquinolone restriction has been associated with a 53% decline in ESBL *Escherichia coli* in Europe.[38] Although these studies suggest ASPs are an effective tool in preventing development of these organisms, once MDROs have developed in a hospital or geographic region, IP initiatives are recommended to prevent further spread[39] and, in fact impact of ASP has been shown to be greater when combined with IP interventions, such as hand hygiene initiatives.[37]

Prevention and management of MRSA bacteremia provide another example of the interplay between IP and ASP to improve the overall care of the admitted patient. IP interventions, such as active screening, contact isolation, and various forms of targeted or universal decolonization, have been studied as ways to prevent transmission of MRSA within hospitals and prevent subsequent infections, including bacteremia.[40–43] When IP preventive efforts fail, *S aureus* bacteremia (SAB) treatment bundles have been effective. Increasing literature now suggests improved adherence to standard of care for SAB may be obtained through implementation of ASP-led bundles targeting timely recommendations of infectious disease consultation, transesophageal echocardiography, source control, follow-up blood cultures, and appropriate, targeted antimicrobial therapy and duration.[44–46]

In our facilities, ASP and IP collaboration on MDRO prevention has primarily focused on CRE control measures and hospital-acquired MRSA tracking and management. For example, beyond day-to-day activities of ASN and IP, when hospital-acquired CRE is identified, ASN pharmacists review past antibiotic history for any missed opportunities while IP examines trends and exposures that may suggest a common source or opportunity for nursing or practice improvement. With regard to MRSA, joint initiatives between IP and ASN have resulted in MRSA screening criteria that capture high-risk individuals for screening so they can be promptly isolated, as well as patients with hospital-acquired pneumonia so antibiotics can be tailored earlier and with more confidence.

SURGICAL SITE INFECTIONS

SSI prevention is another area in which the interplay between ASP and IP can be beneficial in the reduction of infections. Frenette and colleagues[47] saw a 66% decrease in post–cardiac bypass surgery infections with implementation of a combined ASP and IP intervention. Similar bundled interventions using preoperative MRSA screening, targeted decolonization, and targeted preoperative antibiotics resulted in a significant decrease in hip and knee arthroplasty infections and a trend toward decreased cardiac SSIs.[48]

In addition, ASP and IP programs have the opportunity to work together to provide updated guidance for clinicians surrounding the treatment of asymptomatic bacteriuria (ASB) identified via preoperative urine cultures. A recent study by Salazar and colleagues[49] discourages the practice of preoperative screening and treatment of ASB based on findings of no association in the reduction of SSI and urinary tract infections (UTIs) postoperatively.

Evolving literature now suggests the potential of patient-reported penicillin allergies as a contributor to increased risk of SSI due to the receipt of a suboptimal, second-line prophylactic antibiotic agent. According to a recently published retrospective analysis conducted at Massachusetts General Hospital, patients undergoing surgical procedures and concomitantly report having a penicillin allergy had a 50% increased risk of SSI.[50] Although nearly 10% of patients report having a penicillin allergy, in actuality, fewer than 10% of those reporting has a true allergy.[51] This opens the opportunity for preoperative penicillin allergy testing to future endeavors of ASPs to not only improve optimal antibiotic choice, but potentially reduce SSI. ASP involvement with penicillin allergy testing, as well as antibiotic desensitization, is well documented in the literature as a means to ensure appropriate antibiotic utilization and optimization.[52–54]

Similar to interventions mentioned previously, Atrium Health IP staff and ASN pharmacists and physicians have worked together to develop recommendations for preoperative, intraoperative, and postoperative care bundles for colon surgeries to help reduce colon SSIs. Also, IP and ASN physicians have collaborated with surgeons and information services and analytics to develop facility and individual surgeon process and outcome measure performance reports. As SSIs are identified by IP, surgeon and perioperative staff are notified of the infection and any associated fallouts on either antibiotics or colon SSI prevention bundle elements. In addition, facility surgeon-specific SSI scorecards that incorporate cumulative and individual surgeon performance on infection outcomes and process measures are distributed to help foster awareness of data. This work has since spread to hysterectomy and instrumented orthopedic surgeries that are in early stages of implementation.

CLOSTRIDIOIDES DIFFICILE INFECTION

Perhaps one of the most impactful collaborations between ASP and IP programs involve appropriate testing and treatment of CDI. With the rise of toxigenic strains of *C difficile* in the mid-2000s, studies demonstrate that both IP and ASP programs were critical to curtailing the spread of CDI.[55] In a study of CDI outbreak in Canada, implementation of infection control measures was insufficient alone to control an outbreak of nosocomial CDI.[56] Through implementation of ASP interventions to optimize antibiotic utilization in addition to IP measures, CDI rates significantly improved. The "4C antibiotic stewardship" campaign in Scotland similarly demonstrated that a combined intervention of ASP, hand hygiene, and hospital IP significantly decreased national rates of CDI.[9,57]

With the rise of highly sensitive but clinically nonspecific nucleic acid amplification for *C difficile*, diagnostic stewardship initiatives and educational initiatives aimed at clinicians ordering the tests have risen in popularity and necessity.[58,59] Diagnostic stewardship initiatives involving ASP have included a reduction in false-positive hospital-onset CDI through ASP preauthorization and individual clinician education.[60,61]

In our health system, ASP and IP have worked together to improve appropriate ordering of *C difficile* testing and reduced rates of laboratory-identified hospital-onset CDI. This collaboration between IP and ASN included education to both providers and nursing along with joint efforts in the development of an electronic medical record clinical decision support tool that ultimately drives screening and more appropriate testing per an algorithm. The algorithm includes automated alerts for providers who order *C difficile* testing while the patient is on laxatives and/or if the patient does not have a fever or abnormal white blood cell counts around the time of order placement.[62,63] The ASN also focused efforts on the reduction of fluoroquinolone use during daily prospective audit and feedback. Studies such as the one by Shea and colleagues[64] have shown where implementation of a stewardship-initiated respiratory fluoroquinolone restriction program increased appropriate use while reducing overall fluoroquinolones and CDI rates. The combined interventions within the daily workflow of both ASN and IP have resulted in a reduction in hospital-onset CDI within the primary enterprise facilities at Atrium Health.

URINARY TRACT INFECTIONS

More recently, the medical literature reports that inappropriate treatment of ASB and CAUTIs are driving high rates of antibiotic utilization and contributing to the development of MDROs and CDI.[65–67] Newer guidelines and data suggest treatment of ASB is not necessary in most cases.[49,68] ASP educational initiatives have shown reductions in the inappropriate antimicrobial treatment of ASB.[69,70] At 2 Veterans Affairs health systems, a preintervention and postintervention study using a streamlined diagnostic algorithm for CAUTI versus ASB based on IDSA guidelines, along with case-based education for clinicians, showed a significant decrease in overall rate of urine cultures ordered and a significant reduction in overtreatment of ASB.[67]

In our facilities, both ASP and IP have worked together on initiatives to improve appropriate use of urine culture. As one component of a CAUTI prevention initiative, urine culture stewardship education led to a 51% decrease in intensive care unit urine culture ordering with an associated 62% reduction in catheter-associated UTIs.[71] An additional focus for our ASP in 2017 was education around appropriate diagnosis of UTI and treatment of ASB. Inappropriate screening and treatment of ASB has not been associated with decreases in morbidity or mortality but is associated with increased rates of harm and development of multidrug resistance.[69,72] An internal campaign, "Less is More," was designed and implemented for our Atrium Health primary enterprise facilities that equipped our providers with educational tools to help them decide when a patient should appropriately be tested and treated for a UTI.

SUMMARY

ASP and IP programs share more commonalities than differences. Overall goals of both programs are to improve patient safety as it pertains to risk of infection or MDRO acquisition. Although the focus of day-to-day activities is slightly different, the overall themes of surveillance, education, unit rounding, and multidisciplinary interactions are prevalent in both programs. With shared goals, however, comes shared challenges. Achieving sustainable behavior change with constant turnover, information technology issues, being held accountable to a variety of stakeholders, and fighting the never-ending battle to find resources to implement and maintain meaningful programs can seem overwhelming at times. Synergistic work between ASP and IP programs has yielded benefits in prevention of MDROs, SSI, and CDI, as well as reducing inappropriate treatment and testing for ASB. Collaboration between ASP and IP programs can help maximize resources and minimize redundant work to help keep issues related to bugs and drugs at bay.

FINANCIAL DISCLOSURES

All authors have nothing to disclose.

REFERENCES

1. Mcgowan JE, Gerding DN. Does antibiotic restriction prevent resistance? New Horiz 1996;4(3):370–6.

2. Frieden T. Antibiotic resistance threats in the United States. Atlanta (GA): Centers for Disease Control and Prevention; 2013. p. 11–93.
3. The White House. Report to the president on combating antibiotic resistance. 2014. Available at: https://www.cdc.gov/drugresistance/pdf/report-to-the-president-on-combating-antibiotic-resistance.pdf. Accessed March 4, 2019.
4. Obama B. Executive Order – Combating Antibiotic-Resistant Bacteria. 2014;(i):2014-2017. Available at: https://www.cdc.gov/drugresistance/pdf/executive-order_ar.pdf. Accessed March 4, 2019.
5. The White House. National Action Plan for Combating Antimicrobial -Resistant Bacteria.; 2015. Available at: https://www.cdc.gov/drugresistance/pdf/national_action_plan_for_combating_antibotic-resistant_bacteria.pdf. Accessed March 4, 2019.
6. Dellit TH, Owens RC, McGowan JE, et al. Infectious Diseases Society of America and the Society for Healthcare Epidemiology of America guidelines for developing an institutional program to enhance antimicrobial stewardship. Clin Infect Dis 2007;44(2):159–77.
7. Barlam TF, Cosgrove SE, Abbo LM, et al. Implementing an antibiotic stewardship program: guidelines by the Infectious Diseases Society of America and the Society for Healthcare Epidemiology of America. Clin Infect Dis 2016;62(10):e51–77.
8. Centers for Disease Control and Prevention. Core Elements of Hospital Antibiotic Stewardship Programs | Antibiotic Use | CDC. Centers for Disease Control and Prevention. 2017. Available at: http://www.cdc.gov/getsmart/healthcare/. Accessed March 4, 2019.
9. Centers for Disease Control and Prevention. The core elements of antibiotic stewardship for nursing homes CDC. 2017. Available at: http://www.cdc.gov/longtermcare/index.html. Accessed March 4, 2019.
10. Sanchez GV, Fleming-Dutra KE, Roberts RM, et al. Core elements of outpatient antibiotic stewardship. MMWR Recomm Rep 2016;65(6):1–12.
11. Dhar S, Cook E, Oden M, et al. Building a successful infection prevention program: key components, processes, and economics. Infect Dis Clin North Am 2016. https://doi.org/10.1016/j.idc.2016.04.009.
12. Bryant KA, Harris AD, Gould CV, et al. Necessary infrastructure of infection prevention and healthcare epidemiology programs: a review. Infect Control Hosp Epidemiol 2016. https://doi.org/10.1017/ice.2015.333.
13. Scheckler WE, Brimhall D, Buck AS, et al. Requirements for infrastructure and essential activities of infection control and epidemiology in hospitals: a consensus panel report. Infect Control Hosp Epidemiol 1998;19(2):114–24.
14. Bubb TN, Billings C, Berriel-Cass D, et al. APIC professional and practice standards. Am J Infect Control 2016;44(7):745–9.
15. Stone P, Dick A, Pogorzelska M, et al. Staffing and structure of infection prevention and control programs. Am J Infect Control 2009;351–7.
16. Liu H, Herzig CTA, Larson E, et al. Impact of state reporting laws on central line-associated bloodstream infection rates in US adult intensive care units. Health Serv Res 2017;52(3):1079–98.
17. Marsteller JA, Hsu YJ, Weeks K. Evaluating the impact of mandatory public reporting on participation and performance in a program to reduce central line-associated bloodstream infections: evidence from a national patient safety collaborative. Am J Infect Control 2014;42(10):S209–15.
18. Van Santen KL, Edwards JR, Webb AK, et al. The standardized antimicrobial administration ratio: a new metric for measuring and comparing antibiotic use. Clin Infect Dis 2018;67(2):179–85.

19. Moody J, Cosgrove SE, Olmsted R, et al. Antimicrobial stewardship: a collaborative partnership between infection preventionists and health care epidemiologists. Am J Infect Control 2012;40(2):94–5.

20. Abbas S, Stevens MP. The role of the hospital epidemiologist in antibiotic stewardship. Med Clin North Am 2018. https://doi.org/10.1016/j.mcna.2018.05.002.

21. Lou MM, Septimus EJ, Ashley ESD, et al. Antimicrobial stewardship and infection prevention - leveraging the synergy: a position paper update. Infect Control Hosp Epidemiol 2018;39(4):467–72.

22. Monsees EA, Tamma PD, Cosgrove SE, et al. Integrating bedside nurses into antibiotic stewardship: a practical approach. Infect Control Hosp Epidemiol 2019;1–6. https://doi.org/10.1017/ice.2018.362.

23. Kapadia SN, Abramson EL, Carter EJ, et al. The expanding role of antimicrobial stewardship programs in hospitals in the United States: lessons learned from a multisite qualitative study. Jt Comm J Qual Patient Saf 2018;44(2):68–74.

24. Bal AM, Gould IM. Antibiotic stewardship: overcoming implementation barriers. Curr Opin Infect Dis 2011;24:357–62.

25. Pogorzelska-Maziarz M, Gilmartin H, Reese S. Infection prevention staffing and resources in US acute care hospitals: results from the APIC MegaSurvey. Am J Infect Control 2018;46(8):852–7.

26. Haley R, Culver D, White J, et al. The efficacy of infection surveillance and control programs in preventing nosocomial infections in US hospitals. Am J Epidemiol 1985;121(2):182–205.

27. Bartles R, Dickson A, Babade O. A systematic approach to quantifying infection prevention staffing and coverage needs. Am J Infect Control 2018;46(5):487–91.

28. Morris A, Renner-May E, Dalton B, et al. Rationale and development of a business case for antimicrobial stewardship programs in acute care hospital settings. Antimicrob Resist Infect Control 2018;7(104):1–6.

29. Echevarria K, Groppi J, Kelly A, et al. Development and application of an objective staffing calculator for antimicrobial stewardship program in the Veterans Health Administration. Am J Health Syst Pharm 2017;74(21):1785–90.

30. Doernberg S, Abbo L, Burdette S, et al. Essential resources and strategies for antibiotic stewardship programs in the acute care setting. Clin Infect Dis 2018; 67(8):1168–74.

31. Johannsson B, Beekmann SE, Srinivasan A, et al. Improving antimicrobial stewardship the evolution of programmatic strategies and barriers. Infect Control Hosp Epidemiol 2011;32(04):367–74.

32. Wong D, Spellberg B. Leveraging antimicrobial stewardship into improving rates of carbapenem-resistant Enterobacteriaceae. Virulence 2017;8(4):383–90.

33. Snitkin ES, Zelazny AM, Thomas PJ, et al. Tracking a hospital outbreak of carbapenem resistant Klebsiella pneumoniae with whole-genome sequencing. Sci Transl Med 2013;4(148):1–12.

34. National Center for Emerging and Zoonotic Infectious Diseases. Division of Healthcare Quality Promotion. Facility Guidance for Control of Carbapenem-Resistant Enterobacteriaceae (CRE) 2015. Available at: https://www.cdc.gov/hai/pdfs/cre/CRE-guidance-508.pdf. Accessed March 4, 2019.

35. Legeay C, Thepot-Seegers V, Pailhories H, et al. Is cohorting the only solution to control carbapenemase-producing Enterobacteriaceae outbreaks? A single-centre experience. J Hosp Infect 2018;99(4):390–5.

36. Karanika S, Paudel S, Grigoras C, et al. Clinical and economic outcomes from the implementation of hospital-based antimicrobial stewardship programs: a systematic review and meta-analysis. Antimicrob Agents Chemother 2016;60:4840–52.

37. Baur D, Gladstone BP, Burkert F, et al. Effect of antibiotic stewardship on the incidence of infection and colonisation with antibiotic-resistant bacteria and *Clostridium difficile* infection: a systematic review and meta-analysis. Lancet Infect Dis 2017;17(9):990–1001.
38. Sarma J, Marshall B, Cleeve V, et al. Effects of fluoroquinolone restriction (from 2007 to 2012) on resistance in Enterobacteriaceae: interrupted time-series analysis. J Hosp Infect 2015;91(1):68–73.
39. Weiner LM, Fridkin SK, Aponte-Torres Z, et al. *Morbidity and Mortality Weekly Report* vital signs: preventing antibiotic-resistant infections in hospitals-United States, 2014. Morb Mortal Wkly Rep 2016;65(9):235–41. Available at: http://www.cdc.gov/hai/surveillance/nhsn_nationalreports.html. Accessed February 9, 2019.
40. Gidengil C, Gay C, Huang S, et al. Cost-effectiveness of strategies to prevent methicillin-resistant Staphylococcus aureus transmission and infection in an intensive care unit. Infect Control Hosp Epidemiol 2015;36(1):17–27.
41. Traa M, Barboza L, Snydman D, et al. Horizontal infection control strategy decreases methicillin-resistant *Staphylococcus aureus* infection and eliminates bacteremia in a surgical ICU without active surveillance. Crit Care Med 2014;42(10):2151–7.
42. Shitrit P, Gottesman B, Katzir M, et al. Active surveillance for methicillin-resistant *Staphylococcus aureus* (MRSA) decreases the incidence of MRSA bacteremia. Infect Control Hosp Epidemiol 2006;27(10):1004–8.
43. Huang SS, Septimus E, Kleinman K, et al. Targeted versus universal decolonization to prevent ICU infection. N Engl J Med 2013;368(24):2255–65.
44. Ohashi K, Matsuoka T, Shinoda Y, et al. Evaluation of treatment outcomes of patients with MRSA bacteremia following antimicrobial stewardship programs with pharmacist intervention. Int J Clin Pract 2018;72(3):e13065.
45. Smith J, Frens J, Snider C, et al. Impact of a pharmacist driven care package on Staphylococcus aureus bacteremia management in a large community healthcare network: a propensity score-matched quasi-experimental study. Diagn Microbiol Infect Dis 2018;90(1):50–4.
46. Wenzler E, Wang F, Goff D, et al. An automated, pharmacist-driven initiative improves quality of care for *Staphylococcus aureus* bacteremia. Clin Infect Dis 2017;65(2):194–200.
47. Frenette C, Sperlea D, Tesolin J, et al. Influence of a 5-year serial infection control and antibiotic stewardship intervention on cardiac surgical site infections. Am J Infect Control 2016;44(9):977–82.
48. Schweizer ML, Chiang HY, Septimus E, et al. Association of a bundled intervention with surgical site infections among patients undergoing cardiac, hip, or knee surgery. JAMA 2015;313(21):2162–71.
49. Salazar JG, O'Brien W, Strymish JM, et al. Association of screening and treatment for preoperative asymptomatic bacteriuria with postoperative outcomes among US veterans. JAMA Surg 2018;02132:1–8.
50. Blumenthal KG, Ryan EE, Li Y, et al. The impact of a reported penicillin allergy on surgical site infection risk. Clin Infect Dis 2018;66(3):329–36.
51. Joint Task Force on Practice Parameters, American Academy of Allergy, Asthma and Immunology, American College of Allergy, Asthma and Immunology, Joint Council of Allergy, Asthma and Immunology. Drug allergy: an updated practice parameter. Ann Allergy Asthma Immunol 2010;105(4):259–73.e78.
52. Unger NR, Gauthier TP, Cheung LW. Penicillin skin testing: potential implications for antimicrobial stewardship. Pharmacotherapy 2013;33(8):856–67.

53. Jones BM, Bland CM. Penicillin skin testing as an antimicrobial stewardship initiative. Am J Health Syst Pharm 2017;74(4):232–7.

54. Cheon E, Horowitz HW. New avenues for antimicrobial stewardship: the case for penicillin skin testing by pharmacists. Clin Infect Dis 2018. https://doi.org/10.1093/cid/ciy828.

55. Dingle KE, Quan TP, Eyre DW, et al. Effects of control interventions on *Clostridium difficile* infection in England: an observational study. Lancet Infect Dis 2017;17(4):411–21.

56. Valiquette L, Cossette B, Garant M, et al. Impact of a reduction in the use of high-risk antibiotics on the course of an epidemic of *Clostridium difficile*-associated disease caused by the hypervirulent NAP1/027 strain. Clin Infect Dis 2007;45(Supple2):S112–21.

57. Lawes T, Lopez-Lozano J-M, Nebot CA, et al. Effect of a national 4C antibiotic stewardship intervention on the clinical and molecular epidemiology of *Clostridium difficile* infections in a region of Scotland: a non-linear time-series analysis. Lancet Infect Dis 2017;17(2):194–206.

58. Kelly S, Yarrington M, Zembower T, et al. Inappropriate *Clostridium difficile* testing and consequent overtreatment and inaccurate publicly reported metrics. Infect Control Hosp Epidemiol 2016;37(12):1395–400.

59. Polage C, Gyorke C, Kennedy M, et al. Overdiagnosis of *Clostridium difficile* infection in the molecular test era. JAMA Intern Med 2015;175(11):1792–801.

60. Christensen AB, Barr VO, Martin DW, et al. Diagnostic stewardship of *C. difficile* testing: a quasi-experimental antimicrobial stewardship study. Infect Control Hosp Epidemiol 2019;1–7. https://doi.org/10.1017/ice.2018.336.

61. Yen C, Holtom P, Butler-Wu SM, et al. Reducing *Clostridium difficile* colitis rates via cost-saving diagnostic stewardship. Infect Control Hosp Epidemiol 2018;39(6):734–6.

62. Nicholson M, Freswick P, Di Pentima M, et al. The use of a computerized provider order entry alert to decrease rates of *Clostridium difficile* testing in young pediatric patients. Infect Control Hosp Epidemiol 2017;38(5):542–6.

63. White D, Hamilton K, Pegues D, et al. The impact of a comptuterized clincial decision support tool on inappropriate *Clostridium difficile* testing. Infect Control Hosp Epidemiol 2017;38(10):1204–8.

64. Shea KM, Hobbs ALV, Jaso TC, et al. Effect of a health care system respiratory fluoroquinolone restriction program to alter utilization and impact rates of *Clostridium difficile* infection. Antimicrob Agents Chemother 2017;61(6) [pii: e00125-17].

65. Werner NL, Hecker MT, Sethi AK, et al. Unnecessary use of fluoroquinolone antibiotics in hospitalized patients. BMC Infect Dis 2011;11(1):187.

66. Cai T, Nesi G, Mazzoli S, et al. Asymptomatic bacteriuria treatment is associated with a higher prevalence of antibiotic resistant strains in women with urinary tract infections. Clin Infect Dis 2015;61(11):1655–61.

67. Trautner B, Grigoryan L, Petersen N, et al. Effectiveness of an antimicrobial stewardship approach for urinary catheter-associated asymptomatic bacteriuria. JAMA Intern Med 2015;175(7):1120–7.

68. Nicolle LE, Gupta K, Bradley SF, et al. Clinical practice guideline for the management of asymptomatic bacteriuria: 2019 update by the Infectious Diseases Society of America. Clin Infect Dis 2019;1–28. https://doi.org/10.1093/zoolinnean/zly093.

69. Daniel M, Keller S, Mozafarihashjin M. An implementation guide to reducing overtreatment of asymptomatic bacteriuria. JAMA Intern Med 2018;178(2):271–6.

70. Kelley D, Aaronson P, Poon E, et al. Evaluation of an antimicrobial stewardship approach to minimize overuse of antibiotics in patients with asymptomatic bacteriuria. Infect Control Hosp Epidemiol 2014;35(02):193–5.
71. Tyson A, Campbell E, Spangler L, et al. Implementation of a nurse driven protocol for catheter removal to decrease catheter-associated urinary tract infection rate in a surgical trauma ICU. J Intensive Care Med 2018. [Epub ahead of print].
72. Zalmanovici T, Lador A, Sauerbrun-Cutler M, et al. Antibiotics for asymptomatic bacteriuria. Cochrane Database Syst Rev 2015;(4):CD009534.

Collaborative Antimicrobial Stewardship

Working with Information Technology

Kristi M. Kuper, PharmD, BCPS[a,b], Keith W. Hamilton, MD[c],*

KEYWORDS

- Antimicrobial stewardship ● Technology ● Informatics ● Metrics
- Electronic health records ● Clinical decision support systems

KEY POINTS

- Integration of information technology in antimicrobial stewardship programs can improve efficiency and help to scale antimicrobial stewardship interventions.
- Information technology can facilitate administrative tasks of antibiotic stewardship programs, including tracking and reporting antibiotic use data and other metrics.
- Information technology can provide guidance to prescribers at the point of care using clinical decision support and predictive analytics.

BACKGROUND

The earliest reported use of information technology (IT) for the purposes of antimicrobial stewardship was more than 30 years ago when a group of clinicians and researchers used computer algorithms to proactively identify 420 organism-antibiotic mismatches in 1632 hospitalized patients over a 1-year period. Through the use of this technology, they were able to prompt physicians to change or start antimicrobial therapy in one-third of the cases, resulting in improved antimicrobial use.[1] Since this initial article was published, there has been substantial growth in the number of IT programs that have antimicrobial stewardship functionality because of advances in technology, the need to use IT to help meet federal funding requirements (ie, Meaningful Use), and to facilitate compliance with accreditation standards and reporting requirements for antimicrobial stewardship.[2]

The formal application of IT in antimicrobial stewardship is primarily through the use of clinical decision support systems (CDSSs). By definition, CDSSs are electronic tools that are designed to provide intelligently filtered information to clinicians, patient care

[a] Vizient Center for Pharmacy Practice Excellence; [b] DoseMe/Tabula Rasa HealthCare, 228 Strawbridge Drive, Moorestown, NJ 08057, USA; [c] Perelman School of Medicine, Hospital of the University of Pennsylvania, 3400 Civic Center Boulevard, 4th Floor South Pavilion, Philadelphia, PA 19426, USA
* Corresponding author.
E-mail address: keith.hamilton@pennmedicine.upenn.edu

Infect Dis Clin N Am 34 (2020) 31–49
https://doi.org/10.1016/j.idc.2019.10.005
0891-5520/20/© 2019 Elsevier Inc. All rights reserved.

id.theclinics.com

support staff, and patients at appropriate times for the advancement of health and health care.[3] When applied to the management and treatment of infectious diseases, they can assist with identifying patients who require interventions that lead to appropriate antimicrobial use, minimization of toxicity, and improved outcomes.[4,5]

DEFINITIONS

IT support for antimicrobial stewardship programs (ASPs) are primarily facilitated through 4 types of software that use coding and algorithms to prompt a clinical decision: electronic health record (EHR)–based systems, add-on CDSSs, clinical dosing tools, and application (app)-based technology. EHR-based systems (eg, Cerner, EPIC, Meditech) allow all ASP interventions to be performed with a single system. Add-on CDSSs are usually full software-as-a-service programs that can collate data from various sources, produce intervention alerts, and allow intervention documentation separate from the EHR.[6] A listing of selected commercially available add-on CDSSs is available in **Table 1**.

More recently, clinical dosing tools for antibiotics and apps have emerged. Dosing tools, such as *bayesian* dosing software programs, can be used to guide antibiotic dosing in order to maximize the therapeutic benefit of drugs such as vancomycin. These tools may reside within the EHR or exist as a stand-alone system.[7] In addition, apps are increasingly being used to support antibiotic stewardship because of their portability and ease of development and support relative to other IT applications. Apps may be stand-alone, which requires the user to enter patient information, or tethered to an existing EHR-based or add-on CDSS program. An example of the former is an app that provides prescribers a pathway for delabeling and prescribing antibiotics to patients with penicillin allergy labels.[8] The latter allows the autoimport of data into the app, thus reducing the amount of time required by the end user to obtain a result or recommendation.

PATIENT CARE SETTINGS

Each health care setting in which antibiotic stewardship is practiced has unique needs and challenges that can be addressed by IT. These settings include

Table 1
Commercially available add-on clinical decision support systems for antimicrobial stewardship

Product Name	Company (Also Known as)
Bluebird	Intelligent Medical Systems
IC Net	Baxter Healthcare
ILUM Insight	Merck Healthcare Services and Solutions
Lumed	bioMérieux
Medici	Asolva Inc
Patient Event Advisor	BD (MedMined)
PathFinder	Vecna Technologies
RL Solutions	RL Solutions
Sentri 7	Wolters Kluwer (Pharmacy One Source)
TheraDoc	Premier
VigiLanz	VigiLanz

Adapted from Society of Infectious Diseases Pharmacists. AUR vendors. Available at: https://sidp.org/AURvendors. Accessed May 31, 2019; with permission.

hospitals, long-term care facilities, and ambulatory facilities such as clinics, urgent care centers, dialysis facilities, and ambulatory surgical centers. Certain features of IT may be more important in some settings and less important in others. For instance, although the ability to create and customize real-time alerts may be important in hospitals to identify antibiotic stewardship interventions, the ability to perform and customize benchmarking reports and dashboards may be more important in ambulatory facilities. This article addresses some of these unique considerations, but it is important to consider specific needs, goals, and challenges when selecting EHRs, other health care software solutions, and individual IT interventions.

ANTIBIOTIC STEWARDSHIP INTERVENTIONS FACILITATED BY INFORMATION TECHNOLOGY

Daily interventions performed by personnel responsible for antibiotic stewardship are essential to optimize antibiotic use and improve patient outcomes; however, these interventions can be time intensive. IT has the potential to facilitate daily interventions by increasing the scope and efficiency of the ASP. Many daily interventions are most practical in inpatient populations such as acute care hospitals and long-term care facilities, but some may be adapted to ambulatory settings. **Table 2** lists common ASP interventions that can be facilitated by IT.

Table 2
Daily activities for hospital antibiotic stewardship programs that can be facilitated by information technology

Stewardship Activity	Description
Antibiotic time-outs	An antibiotic time-out prompts prescribers to reassess antibiotics at specific times (eg, 48–72 h) when more clinical data are available
Prior authorization	ASPs can restrict use of specific antibiotics that require approval by an ASP team member or infectious diseases specialist
Prospective audit and feedback	ASPs can review antibiotic prescriptions in real time and provide feedback to prescribers on how to optimize antibiotic use based on available clinical data
Automatic stop orders	ASPs can set up automatic antibiotic expiration times (eg, 24 h for surgical prophylaxis) to decrease excess duration of antibiotics
Detection and prevention of antibiotic-related drug-drug interactions	ASPs can monitor for important drug-drug interactions with antibiotics that may limit efficacy of antibiotics or may increase toxicity
Infection-specific and syndrome-specific interventions	ASPs can monitor antibiotic use for specific syndromes that may have high rates of inappropriate antibiotic use (eg, asymptomatic bacteriuria, pneumonia, and skin and soft tissue infections)
Documentation	ASPs must document their interventions to track process metrics and to create a clear record of thought process and recommendations to clinical teams
Communication	Individual patient notes can be left by the ASP team or to communicate information about the patient's therapy from shift to shift or during transitions of care

Antibiotic Time-Outs

An antimicrobial time-out is a defined point in time at which a patient's empiric therapy is reevaluated, usually between 48 and 72 hours.[9] In smaller health care facilities, use of a manual system to track ATOs might be achievable, but is almost impossible in larger facilities where hundreds of patients may be on multiple regimens on any given day unless IT is used. In 2018, Aljefri and colleagues[10] conducted a survey of 71 facilities, and of the 20 hospitals (28%) that had an ATO implemented, 16 used IT to support their ATO programs.

Although many hospitals have implemented or are considering implementing ATOs, data on the use of IT to support these programs and their overall benefit are not well defined. Many of the studies on ATOs have used a paper-based checklist and verbal prompts.[11–13] One study that did engage electronic technology support for an ATO used an electronic checklist embedded in the EHR.[14] Providers seeing patients in a medical intensive care unit (MICU) were instructed to access the checklist when they were reviewing the patients on their daily rounds but received no other verbal or written prompting during the study period. Compared with a second MICU unit, where face to face verbal prompting to conduct an ATO was used, it was less effective in reducing empiric antibiotic use.

Despite the lack of published data showing a benefit, ATO programs are being implemented secondary to suggestions within national guidelines.[15,16] There are multiple ways that IT can be engaged to manage ATOs. The least sophisticated IT approach is to have a report generated from the EHR or add-on CDSS that identifies patients who have been receiving the targeted antimicrobials for the time specified by the ATO policy. Then a designated representative, typically a pharmacist, reviews the list and leaves a note for the prescriber in the EHR notifying the prescriber of a recommended action (eg, stop or de-escalate). In more sophisticated systems, an alert can be built directly into the EHR that is linked to the initial timestamp on the order, and it automatically generates an actionable prescriber alert that can be viewed while managing orders. Rules can be built that can exclude pathogen-directed or chronic prophylactic therapy or fire only for selected antimicrobials in order to reduce alert fatigue. During this process, prescribers may also be asked to specify a total length of definitive therapy, thus potentially minimizing prolonged, unnecessary therapy and creating a second stewardship opportunity. In addition, the intervention action is autodocumented, which can be compiled and reported in monthly ASP statistics.

Prior Authorization

Prior authorization requires several features to implement effectively: (1) a method by which prescribers can contact ASP team members to request the use of restricted antibiotics, (2) a method by which ASPs can respond to providers, and (3) a method by which ASPs can record their recommendations related to the request. IT has the potential to facilitate all of these components. Many ASPs use a phone or pager to facilitate communication between providers and ASP team members. However, CDSSs have been used successfully in other settings to facilitate prior authorization.[17] ASPs could use similar strategies to require prescribers to select appropriate criteria for use through CDSSs using the EHR or clinical surveillance software systems in order to facilitate prior authorization.[18]

This software also has the potential to allow ASP personnel to respond to prescriber requests through the same system, as well as to document their recommendations. Documentation of recommendations is essential to this process to inform pharmacists and the patient care team whether or not the restricted antibiotic should be dispensed.

This documentation can take many different forms, including a note in the EHR by the ASP approver, an electronic message sent to the dispensing pharmacists by the ASP approver, an ASP approver name selected by the prescriber in the antibiotic order, a code provided by the ASP approver entered in the antibiotic order by the prescriber, ASP cosignature of restricted antibiotic orders, or combinations of these strategies.[18,19]

The ideal IT system for prior authorization would create a closed-loop system that could facilitate communication between ASP and prescribers and allow for documentation within the same workflow. In addition, the ideal system would allow for prospective monitoring of the antibiotic before the authorization process to ensure that requests are processed in a timely fashion, that the ASP team does not overlook any antibiotic requests, and that restricted antibiotics are not dispensed inappropriately without ASP approval. In addition, the ideal system would also allow for prospective tracking of antibiotic approval requests so that this information could be reported to track the distribution and approval rate of specific antibiotics and to track the efforts of the ASP to report to administration.

Prospective Audit and Feedback

Prospective audit and feedback can be challenging and inefficient. In any acute care hospital, it is estimated that up to 60% of patients receive an antibiotic per day.[20,21] Up to 70% of residents in long-term care facilities receive an antibiotic over the course of a year,[22,23] and 11% of all residents are on an antibiotic per day.[24,25] Between 30% and 50% of all antibiotic prescriptions in acute care hospitals are inappropriate, and between 25% and 75% of all antibiotic prescriptions in long-term care facilities are inappropriate.[22,23,26] The amount of antibiotic use in larger health care facilities makes manual review of antibiotics impractical because ASPs need to sort through enormous amounts of clinical, laboratory, and microbiologic data to identify potential interventions. In order to make prospective audit and feedback as efficient as possible, ASPs ideally would review only the minimum amount of information to identify situations in which antibiotic use is inappropriate.

Automated alerts have the potential to identify situations in which antibiotic use is more likely to be inappropriate or to need optimization (**Table 3**). These alerts can be created within many EHRs or within add-on CDSSs. Many of these software programs have prebuilt alerts for ASPs. However, some systems require building alerts from scratch or customizing existing alerts to specific patient populations. Partnership with IT staff at health care facilities is often necessary to design or modify these alerts. When considering a new EHR or add-on CDSS, ASPs should evaluate it for (1) compatibility with existing software systems, (2) prebuilt alert infrastructure, (3) customizability, and (4) ease of use.

It is essential to consider compatibility with existing software systems and to inquire whether the software company previously has successfully implemented the software with a hospital's specific software infrastructure, especially with laboratory software and medication ordering and administration software. Different alerts may require data feeds for medication administration and ordering, laboratory and microbiology results, and/or diagnoses and antibiotic indications. If the alert software is not compatible with these data feeds, then alerts may not function properly.

Evaluating prebuilt alert infrastructure is important in order to assess how much effort would need to be placed on creating alerts based on an individual health care facility's needs. Similarly, the ability to customize alerts in the future is important, because new alerts may need to be created or existing alerts may need to be customized.

Table 3
Possible alerts that can be created to facilitate prospective audit and feedback

Alert	Description
De-escalation	Identifies situations in which antibiotic therapy could be narrowed from broader-spectrum antibiotics to more narrow-spectrum antibiotics based on diagnosis, organism identification, or susceptibility results
"Bug"-drug mismatch	Identifies situations in which an organism is identified that is resistant to the active antibiotic regimen
Unlikely infection	Identifies patients on antibiotics without any positive cultures or other diagnostic testing within a defined period of time from initial antibiotic prescription
Inappropriate double coverage	Identifies inappropriate double coverage, including double anaerobic and antifungal drugs
Parenteral to enteral transition	Identifies patients on intravenous agents that are highly orally bioavailable and could be administered orally

In addition, ease of use of alerts is important because the alert system should ideally fit within the work flow of ASP team members. The system of automated alerts also should ideally display relevant clinical, microbiological, and laboratory data to help ASPs sort through information in an efficient fashion without having to toggle back and forth to different clinical systems.[27] Alert systems outside the EHR may be less efficient because chart review and documentation may need to occur in a separate software system from the one that manages alerts. However, systems outside the EHR may be more efficient if they have a more streamlined user interface and/or allow ASP documentation.

Automated alerts can be as simple as alerting the ASP of positive blood cultures or the use of specific antibiotics. They can also be more complex, requiring logic that identifies potential de-escalation opportunities based on diagnosis, microbiological, and antibiotic ordering data. Regardless of the complexity of the automated alert system, prior studies have shown improved guideline adherence, antibiotic use, and patient outcomes when used to facilitate prospective audit and feedback.[27]

An important intersection between new microbiology technology and IT is in the area of rapid diagnostics. Rapid diagnostics such as matrix-assisted laser desorption/ionization time of flight mass spectrometry and multiplex molecular diagnostics have been shown to optimize antibiotic use and improve outcomes.[28,29] Rapid organism identification can allow more expedited ASP notification and intervention. Many rapid diagnostic tests also identify the presence or absence of notable resistance enzymes, creating an opportunity for early streamlining of antibiotics. In order to most effectively leverage rapid diagnostics, IT can alert ASP personnel of these results in real time through the use of electronic alerts so they can help frontline providers to interpret organism identification and the presence or absence of resistance enzymes in order to select the most appropriate antimicrobial therapy.

Automatic Stop Orders

Professional societies have recommended automatic stop orders (ASOs), and some states have mandated them in order to encourage regular review of antibiotics and to prevent unnecessarily prolonged durations.[9] These guidelines and mandates also recommend implementation of some method of informing prescribers when a medication is about to expire to prevent inadvertent stoppages. Common expiration dates for

ASOs include 48 hours, 72 hours, and 7 days. However, some health care facilities vary the ASOs based on antibiotic indication, including providing an exception for pro-phylactic antibiotics.

ASOs have been shown to lead to reduction in antibiotic use and antibiotic-related adverse events in several settings,[30–32] but have shown no difference in others.[33,34] In addition, some studies have reported that ASOs may lead to inadvertent interrup-tion or discontinuation of antimicrobials that are still indicated.[35,36] One study examined adverse outcomes related to a 72-hour ASO and found that approximately 6% of patients had unintended treatment interruptions, although none with clear clin-ical consequences.[35] Therefore, if a health care facility such as an acute care hospital or long-term care facility wishes to create ASOs, engaging IT is crucial in order to implement them in the EHR, to create notifications of expiration to prescribers, and to implement safeguards to prevent adverse events.

Detection and Prevention of Antibiotic-related Drug-Drug Interactions

In addition to reducing inappropriate use of antibiotics and promoting the optimal an-tibiotics, a goal of antibiotic stewardship is to minimize toxicity related to antibiotic use.[9] Antibiotics can interact with a variety of nonantibiotic medications, causing adverse events.[37–40] There are numerous potential antibiotic drug-drug interactions, some more severe and reproducible than others. EHRs include medication interaction alerts in order to notify providers at the time of ordering.

However, prescribers may overlook these alerts inadvertently. Therefore, ASPs may wish to be notified of some potential interactions to help prevent adverse events. IT can facilitate the creation of these alerts within the EHR or using external surveillance software. **Table 4** lists some potential interactions of which ASPs may want to be alerted because of the severity or reproducibility of the reaction, but additional alerts may be added based on the ASP's needs.

Infection-Specific and Syndrome-Specific Interventions

Professional societies and regulatory agencies recommend that ASPs incorporate infection-specific and syndrome-specific interventions as a part of their pro-grams.[9,15,16] The focus of these interventions is to identify and improve prescribing in particular syndromes with potentially high rates of inappropriate antibiotic prescrib-ing, including urinary tract infections, asymptomatic bacteriuria, skin and soft tissue infections, bloodstream infections, and community-acquired pneumonia. Approaches to syndrome-specific interventions may include prospective audit and feedback, ed-ucation, and benchmarking. In larger health care facilities, identifying these syn-dromes by manual review is impractical. However, IT has the potential to more efficiently alert ASPs of potential interventions.

Syndromes that have objective microbiological and laboratory data associated with them could be identified using results from these tests. For instance, positive blood cultures for specific organisms could identify bloodstream infections, and urine cul-tures and urinalyses could identify urinary tract infections and asymptomatic bacteriuria. Automated alerts can be developed based on results of these laboratory tests, and targeting these syndromes has been associated with improved antibiotic prescribing.[27]

However, infections that are not typically defined by culture results, such as pneu-monia and skin and soft tissue infections, may be more challenging to identify because the diagnosis of these infections is based more on clinical characteristics and radio-graphic data. One method of identifying these patients is using the reason for hospital admission. Many inpatient health care facilities code a reason for admission

Table 4
Common clinically significant antibiotic drug-drug interactions

Antibiotic	Interacting Drugs	Clinical Outcome
Carbapenems (ertapenem, imipenem, meropenem)	Valproic acid	All carbapenems reduce plasma levels of valproic acid, decreasing efficacy and increasing risk of seizures
Daptomycin	HMG-CoA reductase inhibitors (ie, statins)	Increases risk of skeletal muscle toxicity
Fluoroquinolones (ciprofloxacin, levofloxacin, moxifloxacin, delafloxacin)	Drugs that prolong the QT interval (eg, antiarrhythmic medications, antipsychotic medications, lithium, methadone, monoamine oxidase inhibitors, and tricyclic antidepressants)	All fluoroquinolones except delafloxacin can cause additional QT interval prolongation, increasing risk of fatal arrhythmias
	Medications or supplements containing divalent cations (eg, antacids, calcium, iron, magnesium, total enteral nutrition, and zinc)	All oral fluoroquinolones: bound by divalent cations, reducing bioavailability and efficacy (separate administration of quinolones by 2–6 h depending on product)
Linezolid	Serotonergic medications (eg, anticonvulsants, antiparkinsonian medications, antipsychotics, dextromethorphan-containing medications, fentanyl, monoamine oxidase inhibitors, selective serotonin reuptake inhibitors, tramadol, triptans)	Linezolid is a serotonergic medication so increases the risk of serotonin syndrome when combined with other serotonergic medications
Macrolides (azithromycin, clarithromycin, erythromycin)	Statins (statins dependent on CYP3A4 for metabolism; eg, atorvastatin and simvastatin)	Clarithromycin and erythromycin strongly inhibit CYP3A4, increasing risk of rhabdomyolysis
	Warfarin	Clarithromycin and erythromycin strongly inhibit CYP3A4, increasing risk of serious bleeding
	Direct oral anticoagulants (eg, apixaban, dabigatran, edoxaban, rivaroxaban)	
	Drugs that prolong the QT interval (eg, antiarrhythmic medications, antipsychotic medications, lithium, methadone, monoamine oxidase inhibitors, and tricyclic antidepressants)	All macrolides can cause additional QT interval prolongation, increasing risk of fatal arrhythmias
	Calcineurin inhibitors (tacrolimus, sirolimus)	Clarithromycin and erythromycin strongly inhibit CYP3A4, increasing risk of calcineurin inhibitor toxicity

Nafcillin	Warfarin	Nafcillin may decrease the anticoagulation effect of warfarin resulting in increased risk of thrombosis; this effect may continue for weeks after discontinuation of nafcillin
Rifamycins (rifampin, rifabutin, rifapentine)	Warfarin	Rifamycins strongly induce CYP enzymes, decreasing anticoagulation effect
	Direct oral anticoagulants (eg, apixaban, dabigatran, edoxaban, rivaroxaban)	Rifamycins strongly induce CYP enzymes and P-glycoprotein, decreasing anticoagulation effect
Tetracyclines (doxycycline, minocycline, tetracycline)	Medications or supplements containing divalent cations (eg, antacids, calcium, iron, magnesium, total enteral nutrition, and zinc)	All oral tetracyclines: bound by divalent cations, reducing bioavailability and efficacy
Trimethoprim-sulfamethoxazole	Warfarin	Sulfonamide antibiotics may increase the anticoagulant effect of warfarin

Abbreviations: CYP, cytochrome P450; HMG-CoA, 3-hydroxy-3 methyl-glutaryl coenzyme A reductase.

This table is not an exhaustive list of antibiotic drug-drug interactions, but includes those commonly encountered in clinical practice. The potential for drug-drug interactions should be determined by searching interactions with drug information software. Most interactions listed in this table are risk rating D (consider therapy modification) or class X (avoid combination) interactions.

electronically. This reason for admission could facilitate identification of specific infections, such as pneumonia and cellulitis, through automated alerts.

Another method of identifying targeted infections or syndromes is by using antibiotic indications. The Centers for Disease Control and Prevention (CDC) core elements for hospitals and nursing homes recommend that all antibiotic prescriptions have a documented indication.[15,41] Many EHRs can be customized to require that an indication be entered with every antibiotic prescription. Especially if prescribers must choose from a selection of discrete indications, these data can be used to alert the ASP when specific antibiotics are prescribed for target indications. In outpatient settings in which prospective audit and feedback are impractical or inpatient settings in which these data are not available electronically, diagnostic coding data could be used to facilitate benchmarking, targeted education, and academic detailing of prescribers.

Documentation

ASPs can document interventions and recommendations in a variety of locations inside and outside the EHR. Although there is variation in the location in which, and the methods by which, ASPs document, the goals are the same: (1) clarify the ASP's role; (2) distinguish sources of clinical information; (3) prompt ASP review of pertinent data that may affect recommendations, such as medication allergies, creatinine, microbiology, and concomitant medications; and (4) document recommendations and the reasoning behind them. Regardless of the location in which the ASP documents, IT can help to facilitate documenting and tracking of interventions. Note that templates have the potential to help standardize ASP review of clinical data by including standard fields and responses (**Fig. 1**). The templates can also import

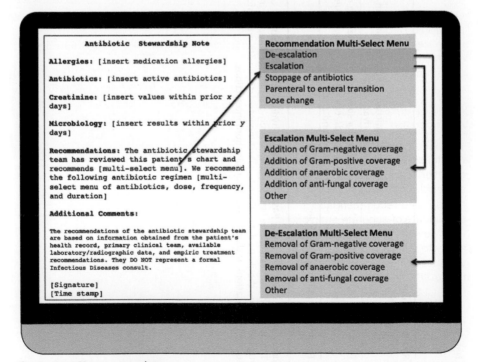

Fig. 1. An ASP note template.

valuable clinical data such as vital signs, allergies, medications, creatinine, and microbiology results as well as include standard disclaimers.

If discrete selections within the note template are stored as discrete data fields, the template could also be used to track the type and frequency of stewardship interventions. This approach would remove the need to document in multiple places in order to track stewardship processes. For instance, the ASP could run or schedule periodic reports to determine the frequency of de-escalation, escalation, antibiotic discontinuation, parenteral to enteral, and dosage change recommendations based on selections within the note. IT may also be able to facilitate tracking of whether or not the clinical care team accepted the team's recommendation in order to track acceptance rates and other stewardship process metrics.

Communication

EHRs and CDSSs can be useful tools to allow communication between ASP team members or individual health care team members (eg, pharmacists) when specific information about a patient needs to be passed from shift to shift. Many of these systems have comment sections that can be used to help communicate current status, intended treatment plan, notes related to communication with other health care providers, or pending drug levels. In some systems, there are also prebuilt note templates that can be used to facilitate communication between a physician and a pharmacist as it pertains to the current antimicrobial therapy and that may be incorporated into the permanent medical record. More recently, some vendors have enhanced their software to allow more real-time communication of alerts or actions needed through texting or instant messaging in a secure format. This ability allows alerts to be pushed to the provider to promote more immediate follow-up on the intervention opportunity. However, other IT clinical systems within the institution may have this type of functionality so it is important to understand what other electronic tools and communication formats are being used. This system helps decrease the redundancy and confusion that can occur with more than 1 communication system in place and can reduce the potential for error or missed opportunities.

AGGREGATE REPORTING, METRICS, AND BENCHMARKS
Antibiograms

Antibiotic susceptibility reports, or antibiograms, are useful for ASPs to track antibiotic resistance, to guide empiric treatment guidelines, and to facilitate empiric antibiotic selection at the point of care. Their creation is recommended by professional societies and public health agencies.[15,41] The Clinical and Laboratory Standards Institute (CLSI) has detailed recommendations on the presentation of antibiograms.[42] Development and update of accurate antibiograms is time consuming when completed manually.

However, IT can facilitate the creation and continual update of antibiograms. The ability to create antibiograms may be available as functionality within an EHR or surveillance software system. If evaluating an automated solution to antibiogram creation, ASPs should obtain the logic used to create the antibiogram to confirm they meet CLSI guidelines.[42]

In addition, some experts have advocated the creation of stratified antibiograms.[42] For example, these may be useful to stratify results by inpatient or outpatient, by groups of unit types, by individual units, by patient characteristics, or by service.[42–44] These stratified analyses can be facilitated and displayed by certain software systems. However, ASPs should use caution when presenting stratified analyses and should put safeguards into place to ensure the number of isolates in each stratification is not less than 30. Small numbers in a given analysis may give misleading results.

Metrics

Present-day IT tools allow easier aggregation of actions and interventions than historical systems such as manual counting or tracking in a spreadsheet. The ability to coalesce massive amounts of transactional data from ASPs has been transformative and has allowed ASP programs to not only justify their resources but also to measure the effectiveness of the program as a whole.

Metrics tracked using IT systems are in 5 general categories (**Table 5**). In some cases, the data originate from a self-contained system, such as within an add-on

Table 5
Antimicrobial metrics that can be tracked using information technology systems

Category	Examples
Antimicrobial use	• DOT or DDD per 1000 patient days • DOT per 1000 patient days present • Percentage of oral therapy • LOT per 1000 patient days • Number of patients on antibiotics (express as percentage of total patients) • Use of individual drugs by MS-DRGs • Antibiotic prescriptions by provider • Average LOT for specific antibiotics • Percentage of visits that result in a prescription (ambulatory care) • New antibiotic starts per 1000 resident days (nursing home setting)
Financial metrics	• Antibiotic cost per patient day or adjusted patient day • Antibiotic cost per discharge • Antibiotic cost per admissions • Cost per MS-DRG • Total cost savings from ASP activities

Process measures	• Interventions by type
	    ○ IV to PO conversion
	    ○ Renal dosing adjustments
	    ○ Antibiotic de-escalation or discontinuation
	    ○ Antibiotic escalation
	• Intervention acceptance rates
	• Average number of interventions per patient
	• Frequency of alerts being generated

Quality and safety	• Adverse drug events reported • Time to appropriate therapy • Time to therapeutic concentrations • Time to PO conversion • Percentage of time that allergies are documented in medical record • Frequency of use of protocols • Compliance to best practice bundles
Outcomes[5]	• Appropriate empiric antibiotic therapy • Resistance rates • *Clostridioides difficile* rates • Length of stay • Readmissions • Mortality

Abbreviations: DDD, defined daily dose; DOT, days of therapy; IV, intravenous; LOT, length of therapy; MS-DRG, medicare severity diagnosis–related groups; PO, oral.

CDSS. In other cases, data need to be combined from multiple systems (eg, her plus financial cost accounting system) or retrieved from a data warehouse. The most common metrics tracked using IT systems are antimicrobial use and interventions. Most IT systems that have antimicrobial tracking capabilities can report use based on days of therapy (DOT) per 1000 patient days. Systems that can track antimicrobial use based on defined daily dose per 1000 patient days are becoming less common, whereas reporting DOT per 1000 days present (the acceptable reporting standard in the National Healthcare Safety Network's antibiotic use module) is becoming more common.

In acute health care settings, antibiotic use is tracked using DOT per 1000 patient days or days present, but, in other health care settings, the use of other metrics may be more useful or more feasible. For instance, in long-term care settings, in which the IT infrastructure may be less robust, it may be more reasonable to generate reports that document number of antibiotic starts per 1000 resident days or list all of the current active antibiotics in the institution, which can be used to conduct a point prevalence study.[41] In the ambulatory setting, the frequency of antimicrobial prescribing by individual prescriber or the percentage of all visits that lead to an antibiotic prescription may be of more value.[45,46]

Financial metrics can be tracked and reported by IT systems, but this ability varies depending on whether or not the system contains or can access financial information. In many cases, the data come from a data warehouse, which is a central location where all of the institutional data from multiple systems is stored and can be retrieved through data queries. Examples of financial metrics may include so-called hard costs, such as overall antibiotic cost savings or costs per Medicare severity diagnosis–related group (MS-DRG). Soft cost savings may be calculated for interventions such as renal dosing or adverse drug reactions prevented. These values are estimated costs associated with the prevention of a potentially negative outcome but do not necessarily translate to a reduction in the facility's bottom line.

Most systems are adept at tracking process measures such as interventions. In some cases, interventions are autodocumented (as previously described) and, in other cases, the individual making the intervention documents it in the system and subsequently documents whether or not the intervention was accepted or declined. Interventions may then be reported in aggregate by pharmacist, shift, clinic location, floor location, or prescriber service. Most IT systems that track and report interventions have the most common ones preprogrammed (eg, de-escalation) and some allow for customization (eg, antibiotic switch in presence of confirmed β-lactam allergy). Examples of other interventions that can be tracked and reported from either a CDSS or EHR include avoidance of duplicate anaerobic therapy, approval of restricted antimicrobials, intravenous to oral conversion, and dose adjustment in renal dysfunction. Almost all IT systems have the ability to generate reports on interventions. These reports are helpful for documenting the frequency that the software is being used and where most of the actionable work is occurring in the system. These reports can be presented at committee meetings, used to justify or support the need for more personnel, or provided to surveyors during accreditation visits as a means to document the work of the ASP or satisfy the request for metrics.

In addition to intervention data, these systems can be useful in identifying the frequency of alerts that are generated, and the metrics generated from these alert reports can be analyzed to identify opportunities for rule refinement and alerting. In 1 study of a 793-bed academic medical center, 48,295 alerts were generated annually for antimicrobials but only 3320 (6.9%) led to a documented intervention.[47] This large gap between identified and actionable alerts resulting in an intervention indicated that opportunities existed to refine the number of alerts that required pharmacist review. These types of reports can identify which stewardship alerts have the highest yield and provide the most return on time investment.

IT systems can also be used to track and monitor ASP quality and antibiotic safety, and clinical outcomes. Metrics generated from an EHR can identify which protocols are being used and with what frequency to determine compliance with institutional best practices for treating certain disease states. McGinn and colleagues[48] evaluated compliance with an evidence-based clinical decision support tool integrated into their EHR for streptococcal pharyngitis and pneumonia. Through their EHR, they were able to determine the frequency with which the tool was used and subsequently found that antibiotic use and rapid streptococcal testing was less when the tool was used versus Not used. Adverse drug reactions (ADRs) and medication safety improvement opportunities can be tracked and analyzed to identify where additional staff education or intervention is needed to reduce their frequency of occurrence. For example, reports can be generated to identify the number of times an alert was generated for a patient that was prescribed a β-lactam in the presence of a penicillin allergy and include the number of times that an intervention was made that could have prevented an ADR. Dosing software programs can identify the frequency with which levels of therapeutic drugs, such as vancomycin, are in the desired pharmacodynamic range,[7] which can be associated with improved outcomes in critically ill patients.[49] Other outcomes that can be measured by IT systems include percentage of length of stay, mortality, and percentage of appropriate empiric antibiotic therapy.[5] EHRs and add-on CDSSs also have the ability to measure and report antibiotic resistance rates and, in some cases, this information can be superimposed graphically over antibiotic use rates to monitor trends. They also have the ability to measure and report the frequency of *Clostridioides* (*Clostridium*) *difficile* rates, which is a metric that can be tied to the success of an ASP[9] and significantly affects patient outcomes.

Periodic Benchmarking

The CDC Core Elements of Antibiotic Stewardship have called for the use of data to facilitate antibiotic stewardship in various health care settings.[15,41,46,50] One way of using data is in the process of periodic benchmarking, or comparing relevant individuals or groups with an accepted standard.[51] ASPs may wish to create regular benchmarking reports with the goal of improving antibiotic prescribing, informing educational efforts, and directing academic detailing. However, these reports can also be used to motivate prescribers to use antibiotics more appropriately. Benchmarking reports could be created on different levels, including individual prescriber, patient care unit, clinic, and health care facility. Some systems only allow the users to access their own data, whereas other systems have the ability to allow the users to benchmark themselves against facilities outside their health system or network, including those in other geographic regions.

In a cluster randomized trial involving an educational and periodic benchmarking intervention throughout a pediatric primary care network, there was a decrease in broad-spectrum antibiotic prescribing and off-guideline prescribing in intervention practices compared with controls.[52] Similar studies in adult primary care practices have yielded comparable results.[53–55] Especially in ambulatory settings, using periodic benchmarking to motivate improvement in antibiotic prescribing practices shows promise where traditional inpatient stewardship interventions, such as prospective audit and feedback, may be impractical.

The basic steps in the process of creating benchmarking data include (1) identifying target benchmarking metrics, (2) extracting pertinent data, (3) displaying metrics in easily interpreted reports, and (4) disseminating reports to relevant parties. IT has the potential to facilitate all components of the benchmarking process. Once target metrics that can be readily extracted from the EHR are identified, IT can be used to set up ongoing data feeds. Depending on available resources, reports can be created within the EHR or by using external analytics or data visualization software platforms. Dissemination of reports to relevant parties can also be facilitated by IT. If reports are displayed within the EHR, dissemination can occur within the EHR in a closed-loop system. If reports are generated via external software platforms, the reports can be disseminated through automated or semiautomated electronic messaging. ASPs should discuss with IT specialists at their health care facilities to determine what methods of data acquisition, display, and dissemination are available if benchmarking is considered.

PREDICTIVE ANALYTICS

The decision to prescribe an antibiotic and the decision of which antibiotics to prescribe are based on a complex series of factors that clinicians must navigate. Much of these decisions are made with incomplete or preliminary data. However, choosing the correct antibiotic is important. Delay in administration of the correct antibiotic in severe infections such as sepsis is associated with significant increases in morbidity and mortality.[56] Patients with very resistant bacteria such as carbapenem-resistant Enterobacteriaceae have mortalities as high as 50%, likely in part caused by not receiving antibiotics in a timely manner.[57] In contrast, choosing an antibiotic that is too broad can expose patients to unnecessary risk of complications such as C difficile infection and adverse drug events, as well as unnecessarily increasing antibiotic resistance.

Predictive analytics are a variety of statistical techniques, including predictive modeling and machine learning, that are used to evaluate present and past data to make predictions about future or unknown events. At some point, predictive analytics may play a key role in antibiotic stewardship by facilitating stewardship processes (eg, prospective audit and feedback, prior authorization, benchmarking, and antibiotic use metrics), identifying target populations, and guiding antibiotic selection to ensure that the right patient receives the right antibiotic at the right time.

Predictive analytics have shown promise in identifying populations at high risk for developing sepsis, resulting in more timely sepsis care.[58] Different approaches have been used for sepsis detection, including clinical risk scores and machine learning.[58–63] Many of these approaches have shown outstanding sensitivity and negative predictive value for the detection of sepsis, but have had variable specificity and positive predictive value. However, the impact on patient outcomes beyond process metrics has been mixed. Additional study is needed to determine clinical outcomes, but predictive analytics have the potential to activate clinical teams to initiate early sepsis care and to alert the ASP to ensure that appropriate antibiotics are selected.

Some antibiotic stewardship software has even shown promising preliminary data by using various real-time predictive analytical techniques to predict antibiotic susceptibility based on patient-specific risk factors available in the EHR. This software has shown outstanding performance characteristics for predicting antibiotic susceptibility.[64,65]

In the future, predictive analytics may become more common in ASPs to target stewardship interventions and to improve empiric antibiotic prescribing decisions. Although not essential components of antibiotic stewardship, predictive analytics can be evaluated as a factor when making decisions about stewardship software. However, additional study is required to determine the clinical outcomes related to predictive analytics.

SUMMARY

The rapid expansion of EHRs and other health care software systems allows the integration of IT for antimicrobial stewardship in a variety of health care settings. Collaborating with IT can improve efficiency and help to scale daily antimicrobial stewardship interventions. IT can also provide guidance to prescribers at the point of care using CDSSs and predictive analytics and can facilitate administrative tasks of antibiotic stewardship programs, including tracking and reporting antibiotic use data and cost savings.

DISCLOSURES

The authors have no disclosures.

ACKNOWLEDGEMENTS

K. Kuper - At the time of initial writing of this manuscript, the author's affiliation was Vizient Center for Pharmacy Practice Excellence. Current affiliation is DoseMe/Tabula Rasa HealthCare, 228 Strawbridge Drive, Moorestown, NJ 08057, USA.

REFERENCES

1. Pestotnik SL, Evans RS, Burke JP, et al. Therapeutic antibiotic monitoring: surveillance using a computerized expert system. Am J Med 1990;88:43–8.
2. Kuper KM, Nagel JL, Kile JW, et al. The role of electronic health record and "add-on" clinical decision support systems to enhance antimicrobial stewardship programs. Infect Conrol Hosp Epidemiol 2019;40:501–11.
3. Office of the National Coordinator for Health Information Technology. Clinical decision support. Available at: https://www.healthit.gov/topic/safety/clinical-decision-support. Accessed May 30, 2019.
4. Pettit NN, Han Z, Choksi AR, et al. Improved rates of antimicrobial stewardship interventions following implementation of the Epic antimicrobial stewardship module. Infect Control Hosp Epidemiol 2018;39(8):980–2.
5. Carracedo-Martinez E, Gonzalez-Gonzalez C, Teixeira-Rodrigues A, et al. Computerized clinical decision support systems and antibiotic prescribing: a systematic review and meta-analysis. Clin Ther 2019;41:552–81.
6. Forrest GN, Van Schooneveld TC, Kullar R, et al. Use of electronic health records and clinical decision support systems for antimicrobial stewardship. Clin Infect Dis 2014;59(Suppl 3):S122–33.
7. Turner RB, Kojiro K, Shephard EA, et al. Review and validation of Bayesian dose-optimizing software and equations for calculation of the vancomycin area under the curve in critically ill patients. Pharmacotherapy 2018;38:1174–83.
8. Blumenthal KG, Wickner PG, Hurwitz S, et al. Tackling inpatient penicillin allergies: assessing tools for antimicrobial stewardship. J Allergy Clin Immunol 2017;140:154–61.
9. Barlam TF, Cosgrove SE, Abbo LM, et al. Implementing an antibiotic stewardship program: guidelines by the Infectious Diseases Society of America and the Society for Healthcare Epidemiology of America. Clin Infect Dis 2016;62:e51–77.
10. Aljefri D, Cruce C, Kinn P, et al. Characterization of antibiotic timeout program strategies across the United States. ID Week, 2018. San Francisco, CA.
11. Thom KA, Tamma PD, Harris AD, et al. Impact of a prescriber-driven antibiotic time-out on antibiotic use in hospitalized patients. Clin Infect Dis 2019;68:1581–4.

12. Lesprit P, Landelle C, Girou E, et al. Reassessment of intravenous antibiotic therapy using a reminder or direct counselling. J Antimicrob Chemother 2010;65:789–95.

13. Lee TC, Frenette C, Jayaraman D, et al. Antibiotic self-stewardship: trainee-led structured antibiotic time-outs to improve antimicrobial use. Ann Intern Med 2014;161(10 Suppl):S53–8.

14. Weiss CH, DiBardino D, Rho J, et al. A clinical trial comparing physician prompting with an unprompted automated electronic checklist to reduce empirical antibiotic utilization. Crit Care Med 2013;41:2563–9.

15. Centers for Disease Control and Prevention. Core elements of hospital antibiotic stewardship programs. Available at: https://www.cdc.gov/antibiotic-use/healthcare/implementation/core-elements.html. Accessed April 11, 2019.

16. The Joint Commission. New antimicrobial stewardship standard. Available at: www.jointcommission.org/assets/1/6/New_Antimicrobial_Stewardship_Standard.pdf. Accessed April 11, 2019.

17. Newcomer LN, Weininger R, Carlson RW. Transforming prior authorization to decision support. J Oncol Pract 2017;13:e57–61.

18. Reed EE, Stevenson KB, West JE, et al. Impact of formulary restriction with prior authorization by an antimicrobial stewardship program. Virulence 2013;4(2):158–62.

19. Dassner AM, Girotto JE. Evaluation of a second-sign process for antimicrobial prior authorization. J Ped Infect Dis Soc 2018;7(2):113–8.

20. Polk RE, Hohmann SF, Medvedev S, et al. Benchmarking risk-adjusted adult antibacterial drug use in 70 US academic medical center hospitals. Clin Infect Dis 2011;53:1100–10.

21. Baggs J, Fridkin SK, Pollack LA, et al. Estimating national trends in inpatient antibiotic use among US hospitals from 2006 to 2012. JAMA Intern Med 2016;176(11):1639–48.

22. Nicolle LE, Bentley DW, Garibaldi R, et al. Antimicrobial use in long-term-care facilities. SHEA Long-Term-Care Committee. Infect Control Hosp Epidemiol 2000;21(8):537–45.

23. Lim CJ, Kong DC, Stuart RL. Reducing inappropriate antibiotic prescribing in the residential care setting: current perspectives. Clin Interv Aging 2014;9:165–77.

24. Centers for Disease Control and Prevention. Antibiotic use in the United States, 2017: progress and opportunities. Available at: https://www.cdc.gov/antibiotic-use/stewardship-report/nursing-homes.html. Accessed April 9, 2019.

25. Nicolle LE, Bentley D, Garibaldi R, et al. Antimicrobial use in long-term-care facilities. Infect Control Hosp Epidemiol 1996;17:119–28.

26. Hecker MT, Aron DC, Patel NP, et al. Unnecessary use of antimicrobials in hospitalized patients: current patterns of misuse with an emphasis on the antianaerobic spectrum of activity. Arch Intern Med 2003;163:972–8.

27. Evans RS, Olson JA, Stenehjem E, et al. Use of computer decision support in an antimicrobial stewardship program (ASP). Appl Clin Inform 2015;6(1):120–35.

28. Huang AM, Newton D, Kunapuli A, et al. Impact of rapid organism identification via matrix-assisted laser desorption/ionization time-of-flight combined with antimicrobial stewardship team intervention in adult patients with bacteremia and candidemia. Clin Infect Dis 2013;57:1237–45.

29. Perez KK, Olsen RJ, Musick WL, et al. Integrating rapid pathogen identification and antimicrobial stewardship significantly decreases hospital costs. Arch Pathol Lab Med 2013;137:1247–54.

30. Tolia VN, Desai S, Qin H, et al. Implementation of an automatic stop order and initial antibiotic exposure in very low birth weight infants. Am J Perinatol 2017; 34:105–10.

31. Murray C, Shaw A, Lloyd M, et al. A multidisciplinary intervention to reduce antibiotic duration in lower respiratory tract infections. J Antimicrob Chemother 2014; 69:515–8.

32. Engels DR, Evans GE, McKenna SM. Effect on duration of antimicrobial therapy of removing and reestablishing an automatic stop date policy. Can J Hosp Pharm 2004;57:214–9.

33. Ross RK, Beus JM, Metjian TA, et al. Safety of automatic end dates for antimicrobial orders to facilitate stewardship. Infect Control Hosp Epidemiol 2016;37:974–8.

34. Do J, Walker SA, Walker SE, et al. Audit of antibiotic duration of therapy, appropriateness and outcome in patients with nosocomial pneumonia following the removal of an automatic stop-date policy. Eur J Clin Microbiol Infect Dis 2012; 31:1819–31.

35. Connor DM, Binkley S, Fishman NO, et al. Impact of automatic orders to discontinue vancomycin therapy on vancomycin use in an antimicrobial stewardship program. Infect Control Hosp Epidemiol 2007;28:1408–10.

36. Cleary JD, Taylor JW, Nolan RL. Automatic stop-order procedure for antibiotics needs evaluation. Am J Health Syst Pharm 1991;48(12):2602–4.

37. Ament PW, Bertolino JG, Liszewski JL. Clinically significant drug interactions. Am Fam Physician 2000;61(6):1745–54.

38. Glasheen JJ, Fugit RV, Prochazka AV. The risk of overanticoagulation with antibiotic use in outpatients on stable warfarin regimens. J Gen Intern Med 2005; 20(7):653–6.

39. Zwart-van Rijkom JEF, Uijtendaal EV, ten Berg MJ, et al. Frequency and nature of drug-drug interactions in a Dutch university hospital. Br J Clin Pharmacol 2009; 68(2):187–93.

40. Wolters Kluwer Clinical Drug Information, Inc. (Lexi-Drugs). Wolters Kluwer Clinical Drug Information, Inc. Available at: https://online.lexi.com/lco/action/login. Accessed April 17, 2019.

41. Centers for Disease Control and Prevention. The core elements of antibiotic stewardship for nursing homes. Available at: https://www.cdc.gov/longtermcare/pdfs/core-elements-antibiotic-stewardship.pdf. Accessed April 11, 2019.

42. Hindler JF, Stelling J. Analysis and presentation of cumulative antibiograms: a new consensus guideline from the Clinical Laboratory Standards Institute. Clin Infect Dis 2007;44(6):867–73.

43. Bosso JA, Mauldin PD, Steed LL. Consequences of combining cystic fibrosis- and non-cystic fibrosis-derived Pseudomonas aeruginosa antibiotic susceptibility results in hospital antibiograms. Ann Pharmacother 2006;40:1946–9.

44. Horvat RT, Klutman NE, Lacy MK, et al. Effect of duplicate isolates of methicillin-susceptible and methicillin-resistant Staphylococcus aureus on antibiogram data. J Clin Microbiol 2003;41:4611–6.

45. Meeker D, Linder JA, Fox CR, et al. Effect of behavioral interventions on inappropriate antibiotic prescribing among primary care practices: a randomized clinical trial. JAMA 2016;315:562–70.

46. Sanchez GV, Fleming-Dutra KE, Roberts RM, et al. Core elements of outpatient antibiotic stewardship. MMWR Recomm Rep 2016;65(No. RR-6):1–12.

47. Hohlfelder B, Stashek C, Anger KE, et al. Utilization of a pharmacy clinical surveillance system for pharmacist alerting and communication at a tertiary academic medical center. J Med Syst 2016;24. https://doi.org/10.1007/s10916-015-0398-9.

48. McGinn TG, McCullagh L, Kannry J, et al. Efficacy of an evidence-based clinical decision support in primary care practices. JAMA Intern Med 2013;173:1584–91.

49. Zelenitsky S, Rubinstein E, Ariano R, et al. Vancomycin pharmacodynamics and survival in patients with methicillin-resistant *Staphylococcus aureus*-associated septic shock. Int J Antimicrob Agents 2013;41:255–60.

50. Implementation of antibiotic stewardship core elements at small and critical access hospitals. Centers for Disease Control and Prevention website. 2017. Available at: https://www.cdc.gov/antibiotic-use/healthcare/implementation/core-elements-small-critical.html. Accessed May 31, 2019.

51. Brotherton AL. Metrics of antimicrobial stewardship programs. Med Clin North Am 2018;102:965–76.

52. Gerber JS, Prasad PA, Fiks AG, et al. Effect of an outpatient antimicrobial stewardship intervention on broad-spectrum antibiotic prescribing by primary care pediatricians. JAMA 2013;309(22):2345–52.

53. Madridejos-Mora R, Amado-Guirado E, Pérez-Rodríguez MT. Effectiveness of the combination feedback and educational recommendations for improving drug prescription in general practice. Med Care 2004;42(7):643–8.

54. Gjelstad S, Høye S, Straand J, et al. Improving antibiotic prescribing in acute respiratory tract infections: cluster randomized trial from Norwegian general practice (prescription peer academic detailing (Rx-PAD) study). BMJ 2013;347:f4403.

55. Meeker D, Knight TK, Friedberg MW, et al. Nudging guideline-concordant antibiotic prescribing: a randomized clinical trial. JAMA Intern Med 2014;174(3):425–31.

56. Gaieski DF, Mikkelsen ME, Band RA, et al. Impact of time to antibiotics on survival in patients with severe sepsis or septic shock in whom early goal-directed therapy was initiated in the emergency department. Crit Care Med 2010;38(4):1045–53.

57. Ben-David D, Kordevani R, Keller N, et al. Outcome of carbapenem resistant *Klebsiella pneumoniae* bloodstream infections. Clin Microbiol Infect 2012;18(1):54–60.

58. Umscheid CA, Betesh J, VanZandbergen C, et al. Development, implementation and impact of an automated early warning and response system for sepsis. J Hosp Med 2015;10(1):26–31.

59. Mao Q, Jay M, Hoffman JL, et al. Multicentre validation of a sepsis prediction algorithm using only vital sign data in the emergency department, general ward and ICU. BMJ Open 2018;8(1):e017833.

60. Liu R, Greenstein JL, Granite SJ, et al. Data-driven discovery of a novel sepsis preshock state predicts impending septic shock in the ICU. Sci Rep 2019;9:6145.

61. Taylor RA, Pare JR, Venkatesh AK, et al. Prediction of in-hospital mortality in emergency department patients with sepsis: a local big data-driven, machine learning approach. Acad Emerg Med 2016;23:269–78.

62. Calvert JS, Price DA, Chettipally UK, et al. A computational approach to early sepsis detection. Comput Biol Med 2016;74:69–73.

63. Horng S, Sontag DA, Halpern Y, et al. Creating an automated trigger for sepsis clinical decision support at emergency department triage using machine learning. PLoS One 2017;12:e0174708.

64. Varga A, Cressman L, Lautenbach E, et al. Use of a precision antibiotic therapy (PAT) prediction model to identify multidrug-resistant Gram-negative organisms. IDWeek 2017; San Diego, CA.

65. Hamilton KW, Cluzet V, Cressman L, et al. Clinical impact of real-time predictive model to facilitate antibiotic prescribing in Gram-negative bacteremia. IDWeek 2018. San Francisco, CA.

Collaborative Antimicrobial Stewardship
Working with Microbiology

Elizabeth L. Palavecino, MD[a], John C. Williamson, PharmD[b,c],
Christopher A. Ohl, MD[c],*

KEYWORDS

- Antimicrobial stewardship • Role of microbiology laboratory
- Infectious diseases diagnosis • Rapid testing • Molecular panels • Antibiogram
- *Clostridium difficile*

KEY POINTS

- The microbiology laboratory should be integrated into antibiotic stewardship programs.
- Rapid diagnostic technologies have the potential of decreasing time to appropriate therapy and improving patient care, and should be implemented in consultation with clinicians, clinical microbiologists, and the antibiotic stewardship team.
- Antibiotic stewardship teams are helpful to guide clinician use of the microbiology laboratory and interpretation of antimicrobial susceptibility results.

INTRODUCTION

Inappropriate and excessive use of antibiotics contributes to the emergence of antimicrobial resistance and adverse patient outcomes including *Clostridium difficile* infection (CDI), adverse drug reactions, and other antimicrobial-related patient morbidities.[1,2] The primary goal of an antimicrobial stewardship program (ASP) is to optimize the appropriate use of antimicrobials, improve patient outcomes, reduce adverse sequelae of antimicrobial use, and decrease the emergence and spread of multidrug-resistant infections.[3,4] The Infectious Diseases Society of America and the Society for Healthcare Epidemiology of America published guidelines in 2007 and updated them in 2016 to assist hospitals to develop and implement ASP and activities.[5,6] Moreover, in 2014 the Centers for Disease Control and Prevention defined seven core elements for successful ASPs,[7] and in 2016 the Joint Commission issued

[a] Department of Pathology, Wake Forest Baptist Health, Winston-Salem, NC, USA;
[b] Department of Pharmacy, Wake Forest Baptist Health, Winston-Salem, NC, USA;
[c] Department of Internal Medicine, Section on Infectious Diseases, Wake Forest Baptist Health, Winston-Salem, NC, USA
* Corresponding author. Section on Infectious Diseases, Wake Forest Baptist Health, Medical Center Boulevard, Winston-Salem, NC 27157.
E-mail address: cohl@wakehealth.edu

Infect Dis Clin N Am 34 (2020) 51–65
https://doi.org/10.1016/j.idc.2019.10.006
0891-5520/20/© 2019 Elsevier Inc. All rights reserved.

id.theclinics.com

regulatory guidance for these programs.[8] These guidelines suggest that ASPs actively collaborate with clinical microbiology.

At Wake Forest Baptist Health (WFBH), an 850-bed tertiary care center with a large cancer center and transplant services, our ASP has been active for 20 years. From the earliest days WFBH's clinical microbiology laboratory director has collaborated with the antimicrobial stewardship (AS) team. This strong partnership between the ASP team and laboratory has been extremely fruitful and has resulted in many successful initiatives to improve patient care. In addition, this collaboration has been helpful to address the challenges of assimilating new outpatient and inpatient clinical facilities into our rapidly expanding health care system. These challenges include finding solutions for the integration of diverse existing susceptibility reporting cascades, infectious diseases testing practices, antimicrobial formularies, and ASPs for newly assimilated hospitals and clinics. In this review, we discuss the collaborative efforts undertaken by our AS team with the microbiology laboratory, illustrating our experience, insight, and some successes and challenges we have encountered.

COLLABORATION WITH THE MICROBIOLOGY LABORATORY

The clinical microbiology laboratory is an essential part of the ASP team and plays an important role in the promotion of appropriate antimicrobial use, surveillance for resistant pathogens, and prevention of nosocomial infections. Conversely, the ASP team is an extremely important entity to advise, support, and expand clinician outreach for the microbiology laboratory. The collaborative tasks between our AS team and the microbiology laboratory include selecting antimicrobial susceptibility testing panels and cascade reporting, reviewing the annual antibiogram, evaluating new methodologies for the diagnosis of infectious diseases, standardizing antimicrobial reporting throughout the health system, educating and communicating with providers, and providing interpretation of test results to guide appropriate use of antimicrobials (**Table 1**). These functions require not only close collaboration of the AS team with the clinical microbiology laboratory, but also the support and expertise of informatics, and hospital leadership, so that providers accept and follow resulting clinical guidance. The acceptance of the recommendations by the clinical providers at large is of the utmost importance for the long-term success of any implemented program or intervention and the AS team can often facilitate such acceptance.

SELECTION OF ANTIMICROBIAL SUSCEPTIBILITY PANELS AND CASCADE REPORTING

Once a year, the ASP staff and the director of the microbiology laboratory review the current antimicrobial susceptibility panels and the corresponding set of tested antimicrobials. Updated panel contents are reviewed focusing on the addition of new agents or the modified antimicrobial concentrations that are tested that may be relevant to our specific treatment guidelines. To ensure that the laboratory is providing the most clinically relevant antimicrobial susceptibility results, our program routinely validates and implements new breakpoint recommendations from the Clinical and Laboratory Standards Institute (CLSI).[9]

In addition to the standard rules for cascade reporting recommended by CLSI,[9] our program developed additional rules for antimicrobial susceptibility reporting so that results for some agents are "hidden." Hidden susceptibilities are often agents that would be problematic for treating selected infections (such as fluoroquinolones for invasive *Staphylococcus aureus*). This facilitates a final goal of promoting the use of the right agent for the right patient. A "hidden" susceptibility result must be approved

Table 1
Main collaborative efforts between the AS team and the microbiology laboratory at WFBH

Efforts/Tasks	Comments
Selecting antimicrobial susceptibility testing panel for routine testing	At least once a year the current panels are reviewed to assess where changes are needed
Review of the reporting cascade	To ensure that the agents reported are included in our formulary and are the preferred agents for treatment
Preparation of cumulative susceptibility reports (antibiogram)	Annual reports are prepared for the different services within the main hospital and for the hospitals in our health care system
Standardization of agents in formulary and reporting of antibiotics throughout the health care system	Because the results are entered in the same electronic system, it is important to have the same rules and recommendations for reporting
Assessment of rapid diagnosis tests	Selection of tests is done to maximize clinical usefulness
Deciding what new agents can be available to testing and when to use them	Provide recommendations for testing of newer agents not included in panels, but that can be tested by other methods
Providing interpretation of microbiology tests and cultures	Adding comments to reports to facilitate interpretation
Diagnostic stewardship	Identify areas that need clarification for ordering, collection, or change in methodology to avoid misuse of antibiotics
Education to providers	Multiple options for education including laboratory rounds

by the ASP member on call (or a consulting infectious diseases provider) before the microbiology laboratory can report the results for that agent in the electronic medical record. This reporting algorithm has guided providers to select an agent from among those reported, which are usually of narrow spectrum or enhanced efficacy, or are considered first-line therapy for the organism isolated. Some of our reporting rules for antimicrobial susceptibility results are described in **Table 2**.

PREPARATION OF ANTIBIOGRAMS

An antibiogram or cumulative susceptibility report is the summary of the local rate of antimicrobial susceptibility for the organisms most frequently isolated from clinical specimens. The antibiogram serves as a resource for clinicians choosing empiric antibiotic therapy. By tracking changes in the antibiogram year after year, the antibiogram helps stewardship programs to identify emerging resistance or to document improvements in susceptibility rates after targeted interventions. The microbiology director has traditionally been responsible for preparing and validating the data for the annual antibiogram according to the rules described in the CLSI M-39 document.[10]

Stewardship personnel, including pharmacists, have a vested interest in the antibiogram because of its potential impact on antibiotic prescribing. For this reason, stewardship pharmacists often work with the microbiology laboratory to populate

Table 2
Examples of reporting rules to influence antibiotic decisions

Rule	Rationale
Daptomycin tested but not reported for staphylococci and enterococci	Promote antibiotic stewardship
Linezolid reported for respiratory cultures of *Staphylococcus aureus* but not blood cultures	
Ceftaroline tested but not reported	
Cascaded reporting of linezolid for enterococci (only reported if vancomycin resistant)	
Cascaded reporting of cefepime and ceftazidime for Enterobacteriaceae (only reported if ceftriaxone resistant)	
Cascaded reporting of aminoglycosides for gram-negative rods	
Trimethoprim/sulfamethoxazole reported for wound cultures of *S aureus* but not blood cultures	Prevent inappropriate treatment
Fluoroquinolones and rifampin tested but not reported for staphylococci	
Tetracycline reported for wound and urine cultures but not blood cultures	
Perform D-test for staphylococci and streptococci that are erythromycin resistant and clindamycin susceptible	
β-Lactams not reported for oxacillin-resistant staphylococci	

susceptibilities, validate the data, and format the antibiogram so it is user (clinician) friendly. Color coding can help designate certain antibiotics as preferred based on enhanced susceptibility. Some institutions also add relative antibiotic cost information to the antibiogram to further assist clinicians at the point of antibiotic prescribing.

Modern health care systems are often challenged with standardizing antibiograms to serve many stakeholders within the system. The system's stakeholders include staff working in different settings, such as clinics, nursing homes, long-term care facilities, community hospitals, and tertiary care medical centers. Developing antibiograms that serve each of these settings is difficult. It is important to identify stewardship staff or liaisons at each location who can provide the local perspective about the patient populations served, the antibiotic formulary, the most common infections encountered, and any resistance concerns.

Depending on the structure of the health system, it may be advantageous to consolidate antibiogram data for multiple system locations, especially if the locations have common characteristics (eg, community hospitals or clinics in the same geographic area). Consolidating antibiogram data can also improve the sample size for organisms that are infrequently cultured. However, there are barriers in developing antibiograms to serve multiple locations in a health system. It is possible that different locations use different assays for susceptibility testing or that the antibiotics tested are different because of inconsistent formularies. By working with microbiology, a system stewardship program can help standardize and align these processes, making consolidated antibiograms feasible and improving consistency in the use of antibiotics throughout the system.

Antibiograms are limited in that they provide single antibiotic-pathogen pair susceptibility rates. The adequacy of any single agent prescribed as empiric therapy may not be acceptable in clinical practice, particularly for life-threatening infections among patients with risk factors for antibiotic-resistant bacteria. The addition of a second antibiotic can improve adequacy of empiric therapy, and the optimal combination of antibiotics should be directed by local microbiology data. Specifically, microbiology and stewardship personnel should work together to construct combination antibiograms that represent institution-specific bacterial pathogens for a particular disease and ultimately to determine recommendations in local empiric treatment guidelines, as our team has successfully done.[11]

IMPLEMENTATION OF RAPID TECHNOLOGIES FOR THE DIAGNOSIS OF INFECTIOUS DISEASES

New diagnostic techniques, a rapid turnaround time for pathogen identification, and accurate interpretation of susceptibility results are important tools for a patient-centered selection of appropriate therapy. Throughout the years, our AS team has reviewed many new laboratory techniques and methodologies that allow rapid identification of organisms and their mechanisms of resistance. The local assessment of clinical usefulness of these tests for our patient population has been an important factor for hospital administration in their decision to acquire a new piece of equipment testing methodology. Some of the most relevant technologies for rapid testing in the microbiology laboratory that have been evaluated and implemented by our AS team are described next.

Matrix-Assisted Laser Desorption/Ionization Time-of-Flight Technology for Identification of Organisms

There is no doubt that matrix-assisted laser desorption/ionization time-of-flight (MALDI-TOF) has revolutionized the way that laboratories identify microorganisms. This technique identifies an unknown organism by analyzing the proteins present, separating them according to mass, charge, and the time it takes for each of the proteins to travel from the inoculation site to the detector end of the instrument. Based on these parameters, the instrument generates a protein spectrum that is then compared with the spectrums included in the database of the instrument.[12,13] The main advantages of MALDI-TOF are the speed and accuracy for identifying microorganisms. The instruments have high performance characteristics and robust databases to identify the most common organisms isolated from clinical specimens.[14] Overall, identification is achieved 2 to 24 hours earlier for gram positives, and 24 to 72 hours earlier for gram-negative rods and yeasts compared with traditional systems of identification.[13,15] Furthermore, MALDI-TOF is able to accurately identify fastidious or difficult to identify organisms that laboratories were previously unable to identify with conventional identification methodologies. The reporting of unusual organisms that are occasionally identified by MALDI-TOF can have unintended consequences because clinicians may be unfamiliar with the organism reported or with their potential pathogenicity and this can potentially lead to unnecessary antimicrobial treatment. Consultation with our ASP team is recommended for assessment of reporting language in the medical record and how clinicians might respond to a *Staphylococcus epidermidis* result as compared with a "coagulase-negative staphylococcus" report. Studies have shown that rapid identification of an organism by MALDI-TOF can improve time to appropriate antibiotic treatment, but only when associated with ASP collaboration.[16-19]

The laboratory at WFBH implemented MALDI-TOF technology in 2014 and our AS team has been fundamental in educating providers on how to use the early identification result to implement empiric therapy by providing reliable local antibiogram reports. Overall at our institution, the implementation of MALDI-TOF has clearly improved turnaround time for identification of organisms. Although MALDI-TOF does not provide susceptibility testing, many organisms have predictable susceptibility, and in these cases, rapid identification results in appropriate patient management.

Multiplex Molecular Assays

For many years, molecular detection of a single organism, such as methicillin-resistant S aureus, has shown its clinical usefulness for a single-drug-resistant organism.[20,21] In the last decade, however, there has been a dramatic increase in the development of multiplex molecular assays designed to detect multiple pathogens associated with an infectious syndrome rather than one specific organism. These multiplex polymerase chain reaction (PCR) assays are usually offered as a "panel," which can simultaneously detect, in a single specimen, the pathogens most commonly associated with an infectious syndrome, such as bloodstream, meningitis/encephalitis, respiratory, or gastrointestinal infections.[22]

The implementation of rapid methods must be critically evaluated considering test volume, patient population, and availability of laboratory personnel and clinical support to ensure that the diagnostic technology selected is appropriate for the clinical service at a particular institution. Overuse or inappropriate use of these rapid tests may increase costs without providing the expected improvements in diagnosis and patient care.[23] In addition, many multiplex tests are not reimbursed by third-party payers in the outpatient setting, which can lead to serious economic consequences for the health care system and patient. ASPs affiliated with the clinical laboratory are of value to determine whether test parameters, such as sensitivity, specificity, and positive and negative predictabilities, are useful for implementation. In addition they can help develop protocols that identify appropriate patients for testing and subsequent test interpretation.

(Table 3) describes selected molecular panels that we have implemented and our experience with their use. This table also shows a description of the requirements for ordering these molecular panels.

Blood culture identification panels

One of the most important factors influencing treatment outcomes of patients with bloodstream infections is appropriateness of early antimicrobial therapy.[24,25] In addition to the prompt initiation of effective therapy, avoidance of unnecessary exposure to broad-spectrum antibiotics is important to limit adverse events and prevent the emergence of antibiotic resistance. The main advantage of rapid blood culture identification panels is that they identify the organism 1 to 3 hours after the blood culture has signaled positive compared with 24 to 48 hours using traditional methodologies. Furthermore, these panels can also identify genetic elements of resistance mechanisms, making them useful for selecting antibiotic therapy for multidrug-resistant organisms.[22,26]

At WFBH, we implemented the Biofire FilmArray Blood Culture Identification Panel (BioMerieux, Durham, NC), but because of current resource allocation do not use this panel for all blood cultures. To optimize cost-effectiveness and target patients at greatest risk, we elected to use this test routinely only for blood cultures from patients located in an intensive care or oncology units. We studied the impact of panel implementation for patients with noncontaminant gram-positive bacteremia and found improvements in AS metrics as shown in Fig. 1. These improvements were attributed to

Table 3
Requirements for ordering multiplex molecular panels and comments included in report to facilitate interpretation

Panel	Requirement/Recommendations for Ordering	Comments
RVP	Recommended in immunosuppressed patients with high risk for respiratory complications, and patients with severe respiratory infections that need to be admitted	No test of cure, no repeats of negatives unless new symptoms Encourage no testing or use the rapid flu test if influenza is suspected
GIP	Community-acquired diarrhea of ≥ 7 d duration, travel-related diarrhea, severe presentation (bloody diarrhea, dehydration), immunocompromised status, or norovirus suspected	No test of cure, no repeats of negatives The following comment is included in each report: "No antimicrobial therapy is recommended for mild illness with symptoms <7 d"
MEP	High suspicion of infectious meningitis/encephalitis CSF with signs compatible with infectious process and at least 50 WBCs	If suspecting HSV, order the stand-alone HSV, which has higher sensitivity Culture must be ordered at the same time Likelihood of false positive, correlate with other tests and clinical presentation

Abbreviations: CSF, cerebrospinal fluid; GIP, gastrointestinal panel; HSV, herpes simplex virus; MEP, meningitis/encephalitis panel; RVP, respiratory viral panel; WBC, white blood cells.

the shortened time to organism identification and the ability to detect resistance. Median time to identification improved by 29 hours. Implementation of the panel also improved stewardship metrics for patients with blood cultures positive with a likely contaminant. For patients with blood culture contaminants, our study demonstrated a reduction in days of antibiotic therapy, shorter length of hospital stay, and fewer tests for vancomycin levels.

Optimal use of rapid diagnostic tests, including multiplex molecular blood culture panels, is best done in conjunction with dedicated stewardship personnel who provide

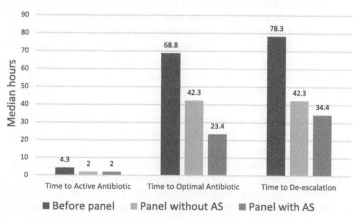

Fig. 1. Impact of a rapid blood culture panel with or without antibiotic guidance on stewardship metrics for noncontaminant gram-positive bacteremia.

antibiotic guidance at the time results are available.[27-31] At WFBH, the AS team and microbiology staff collaborated to evaluate an approach for communicating positive blood culture panel results. Instead of reporting positive cultures to the nurse, results were reported directly to a stewardship pharmacist who relayed the result to the responsible provider along with antibiotic guidance. This method of communicating positive cultures improved stewardship metrics beyond what the rapid panel could achieve alone (see **Fig. 1**).

Some hospitals, however, may struggle to maintain this model of reporting 24 hours a day, 7 days a week. After initial implementation of molecular blood culture testing with AS team reporting, we later elected to report results using in-basket functionality within the electronic medical record in conjunction with traditional reporting to nurses. Inpatient acute care pharmacists received the in-basket results instead of a dedicated stewardship pharmacist. Such passive reporting of panel results did not achieve the same improved stewardship metrics. Time to optimal therapy and time to de-escalation regressed back to levels close to the traditional method of only reporting to nurses (data not shown). Our experience highlights the need for dedicated stewardship personnel along with rapid diagnostics to achieve the best outcomes.

Respiratory viral panels

Respiratory tract infections are one of the most common causes of morbidity and mortality in all age groups, and the clinical presentation of different organisms are often similar. Furthermore, a large portion of lower respiratory tract infections is caused by viruses, mycoplasma, and chlamydophila. A multiplex PCR for respiratory viruses and difficult-to-culture bacteria, including pertussis, is now a frequently used panel test for respiratory infections. Testing for respiratory viruses other than influenza is controversial because many argue that detecting viruses for which there is no treatment may not be clinically important. Others state that identifying noninfluenza respiratory viruses is beneficial because it decreases additional testing, provides valuable information for epidemiologic and infection prevention purposes, and limits the use of antibiotics.[32]

At WFBH, the first respiratory viral panel (RVP), a multiplex PCR for respiratory viruses, was implemented in 2009 around the time of the 2009 H1N1 influenza A pandemic. Initially it was mostly used for the diagnosis of influenza, but it quickly became a useful tool for assessing patients with other respiratory infections. Currently, the laboratory uses a multiplex PCR assay that includes 15 respiratory viruses and four bacterial pathogens. To begin with, microbiology and stewardship staff positioned the RVP for use in immunocompromised patients or those with moderate to severe respiratory infections needing hospitalization. Tests could be ordered without preauthorization or other restriction. Over time, the volume of ordered RVPs has substantially increased, with the maximum volume observed during the months of influenza activity. The high cost of the test and escalating RVP volume underscores the importance of diagnostic stewardship and prudent use of this test. In addition, test performance depends on collecting proper nasopharyngeal swabs and physicians and nurses should be trained on the procedure.

To evaluate whether RVP testing improved stewardship metrics at WFBH, microbiology and stewardship staff collaborated to determine the impact of RVP testing on the use of antibiotics for respiratory infections. We conducted a prospective study of nonimmunocompromised inpatients tested with the RVP and measured antibiotic use associated with respiratory infection. Results of the study showed that providers were more likely to discontinue or de-escalate antibiotics if the RVP is positive

(Table 4). Hospital length of stay and attributable mortality was not changed. Microbiology and stewardship teams need to balance improved stewardship metrics associated with the test with its cost and high volume burden to the laboratory. Thus, although the escalating cost of RVP testing is concerning, it may be offset by reduced antibiotic expense and improved use. At WFBH the stewardship team is currently implementing diagnostic stewardship for the RVP to decrease the volume and improve the selection of patients for testing.

Gastrointestinal panels

Infectious diarrhea is caused by bacterial, viral, and parasitic pathogens and remains a significant health care burden worldwide.[33] Although gastrointestinal infections are severe in immunosuppressed, pediatric, and elderly patients, most of these infections are self-limiting and do not need antimicrobial treatment.[34] Conventional testing for gastrointestinal pathogens lacks sensitivity and takes 3 to 5 days for the results to become available. With the gastrointestinal panels, results are available in 2 to 3 hours and it can detect the most important bacterial, parasitic, and viral pathogens causing diarrhea in the United States. Because the results are available the same day that the sample is submitted, the patient is still symptomatic and this may lead to antibiotic treatment. For that reason, at WFBH, a comment is included with each gastrointestinal panel result with recommendations to prevent misuse of antibiotics. Questions on whether treatment is necessary, such as for positive tests for enteropathogenic *Escherichia coli*, are referred to the stewardship pager.

In addition to improving diagnostic accuracy, this assay has helped us to quickly detect and control norovirus outbreaks as well as a *Salmonella* spp outbreak involving multiple counties in our region.

Meningitis/encephalitis panel

This panel from BioFire can rapidly detect the pathogens most commonly associated with this syndromic infection. However, the published evaluation of the performance of this panel showed false positives particularly for *Streptococcus pneumoniae*.[35] A false-positive result may not only lead to unnecessary therapy, but more importantly, false-positive results may delay or halt the pursuit of the true diagnosis.[36] In addition, providers should be aware that the sensitivity for detection of the different pathogens included in the panel varies considerably. For this reason, at WFBH when suspecting herpes simplex virus (HSV) infection,

Table 4
Impact of RVP testing on antibiotic use at WFBH

Outcome	Negative RVP (n = 100)	Positive RVP[a] (n = 50)	P Value
Antibiotic discontinued by 24 h, n (%)	2 (2)	5 (10)	.04
Antibiotic de-escalated by 24 h, n (%)	8 (8)	13 (26)	<.01
Antibiotic DOT, median (range), d	9 (1–35)	6 (1–53)	.03
Antibiotic duration, median (range), d	4.1 (0.5–14.9)	3.5 (0.2–24)	.09
Length of hospitalization, median (range), d	4.3 (0.4–39.9)	3.6 (0.9–26.0)	.25
In-hospital mortality, n (%)	3 (3)	2 (4)	.75

Abbreviation: DOT, days of antibiotic therapy.
[a] Viruses detected by RVP include influenza (38%), respiratory syncytial virus (20%), metapneumovirus (20%), rhino/enterovirus (18%), and coronavirus (4%).

particularly in neonates, we recommend ordering the stand-alone HSV PCR test in cerebrospinal fluid, which has higher sensitivity than the HSV target included in the meningitis/encephalitis panel (MEP). The main benefit of the MEP is the rapid result, which could help to select appropriate therapy and prioritize resource use. In addition, it has been useful for the determination of whether droplet isolation or secondary chemoprophylaxis is required for *Neisseria meningitis*. Because of the potential for false-positive results and the possibility for the detection of latent or reactivated viruses, results from MEP must be carefully assessed. At WFBH, MEP orders are not routinely processed on specimens with less than 50 WBC/dL unless approved by a consulting infectious disease or AS team member. All positive results for bacterial pathogens are correlated with culture to confirm the diagnosis.

DIAGNOSTIC STEWARDSHIP

Diagnostic stewardship refers to the appropriate use of laboratory testing to guide patient management and treatment in real time, with the goal of enhancing clinical outcomes and limiting the spread of antimicrobial resistance.[37] The goals of the ASP and the microbiology laboratory are intertwined, inasmuch as laboratory results direct antibiotic decision making. All phases of the diagnostic effort, the preanalytical phase, the analytical phase, and postanalytical phase, are critical elements of the testing process because they significantly impact diagnostic accuracy and the antimicrobials prescribed in response to test results.[38] Overuse of unnecessary testing increases the likelihood of false-positive test results that may lead to erroneous diagnoses and inappropriate antibiotic usage. Therefore, the ASP and microbiology laboratory must collaborate to design diagnostic stewardship processes aimed at achieving collective goals. At WFBH, the ASP and microbiology laboratory identified areas that could benefit from diagnostic stewardship. One of our most successful initiatives involves testing for CDI.

Testing for Clostridium difficile Infection

The enzyme immunoassays (EIA) to detect the presence of toxins were initially the most commonly used tests for the diagnosis of CDI, but their low sensitivity resulted in false-negative results. In 2009, WFBH converted to nucleic acid amplification test (PCR) for the diagnosis of CDI and observed a two-fold increase in the number of diagnoses. Growing concerns regarding overdiagnosis of CDI led us to evaluate CDI diagnoses at WFBH in 2015. Clinical specimens submitted for PCR testing were tested concurrently with an EIA that simultaneously tests for *C difficile* antigen and toxin. Members of the ASP performed chart review for each patient and made assessments of the likelihood of CDI while blinded to the EIA results. The analysis showed that the EIA was a better predictor of CDI and confirmed our suspicion of overdiagnosis by using PCR alone. The evaluation also identified common reasons for diarrhea that led to unnecessary CDI testing, many of which were iatrogenic. Several initiatives to improve patient selection for testing and the pretest likelihood for CDI were not successful. These included electronic medical record best practice advisories or algorithms, and nurse and provider education.

Supported by the data in our assessment, we converted to EIA testing in April 2016, ahead of guidelines by European and American societies that recommend a high-sensitivity EIA assay as a first step followed by a high-specificity toxin test.[39,40] Included in the report for each EIA result, we added an explanatory comment (**Table 5**) for clinical decision support. PCR testing is still available at WFBH, but

Table 5
Clinical decision support for interpretation of *Clostridium difficile* EIA results

Result Combination	Interpretation and Comment
Antigen positive, toxin positive	Interpretation: Positive for toxigenic *C difficile*. Comment: These results are consistent with *C difficile* infection. Detection of both antigen and toxin are expected when *C difficile* infection is present.
Antigen positive, toxin negative	Interpretation: *C difficile* present but toxin not detected. Comment: This pattern is most consistent with *C difficile* colonization (occurs in 20% of hospitalized patients). There is no indication to treat *C difficile* colonization and anti–*C difficile* antibiotics do not prevent subsequent infection. Antimicrobial therapy and proton pump inhibitors should be avoided. Consideration should be given to medication causes of diarrhea, such as laxatives, stool softeners, colchicine, metformin, HIV protease inhibitors, antibiotics, or certain chemotherapy agents, among others. Enteral feeds are also a common cause of diarrhea. If symptoms and signs are consistent with colitis and risk factors are present for *C difficile* (eg, recent antibiotic exposure), additional testing using *C difficile* PCR may be performed, but testing requires prior authorization by the AS team.
Antigen negative, toxin positive	Interpretation: Undetermined. Comment: Toxin positivity should not occur without antigen positivity. Consider repeat testing if clinically indicated.
Antigen negative, toxin negative	Interpretation: Negative for toxigenic *C difficile*. Comment: There is no evidence of *C difficile* infection. Consider other causes of diarrhea. Consideration should be given to medication causes of diarrhea, such as laxatives, stool softeners, colchicine, metformin, HIV protease inhibitors, antibiotics, or certain chemotherapy agents, among others. Enteral feeds are also a common cause of diarrhea.

Abbreviation: HIV, human immunodeficiency virus.

requires authorization by a member of the ASP. After changing the assay, PCR testing frequency declined by 98%, the rate of International Classification of Diseases-9/10 codes for CDI declined by 65%, the rate of NHSN *C difficile* LabID event rates/ 10,000 patient days declined by 75%, and the number of patients treated with oral vancomycin declined by 58%. Postimplementation audits showed no increase in CDI morbidity or mortality, or missed cases of inpatient CDI.

Interpretation of Antimicrobial Susceptibility Results

Through the years, we have identified certain antimicrobial susceptibility results that are misinterpreted by clinicians. Such misinterpretation leads to additional but unnecessary testing (eg, "special MIC") or use of alternative antibiotics. The AS team and microbiology laboratory have developed supporting guidance incorporated within test results to overcome these issues. Examples of comments included in test results

Table 6
Examples of comments included in the antimicrobial susceptibility testing report

Organism/Specimen	Comment
Haemophilus influenzae isolated from sterile sites	*H influenzae* is considered susceptible to ceftriaxone and meropenem even if β-lactamase positive.
H influenza and *Haemophilus parainfluenza* from respiratory specimens	*H influenzae* may produce β-lactamase, which causes resistance to penicillin, ampicillin, and amoxicillin. However, *H influenzae* is generally susceptible to amoxicillin-clavulanate, cefuroxime, cefpodoxime, cefdinir, ceftriaxone, and azithromycin even if β-lactamase positive.
Group B streptococcus from vaginal/rectal swab for screening pregnant women	Group B streptococci are universally susceptible to ampicillin, penicillin, and cefazolin and testing is not necessary. If the clindamycin is reported as susceptible, the result has been confirmed by D test, and the organisms should be considered susceptible to clindamycin.
Escherichia coli, *Klebsiella pneumoniae*, and *Proteus mirabilis* from clean-catch urine Cefazolin breakpoints for urine are applied	In the treatment of uncomplicated urinary tract infections, cefazolin susceptibility predicts susceptibility to the oral cephalosporins cephalexin, cefuroxime, cefpodoxime, and cefdinir. Cephalexin is cost-effective, but QID dosing (normal renal function) is less convenient than the other oral cephalosporins, which are dosed BID. Isolates resistant to cefazolin but susceptible to ceftriaxone may be susceptible to cefpodoxime.
Carbapenem-resistant enterobacteriaceae	Based on additional testing the following comment is added: carbapenamase-producing organism. Consult AS team for treatment recommendations.

are listed in **Table 6**. Furthermore, special or extrasusceptibility testing must be approved by a member of the AS team.

SUMMARY

Rapid methodologies, particularly multiplex molecular panels, represent a paradigm shift in the diagnosis of clinical infectious diseases. The main benefit of rapid assays is the potential for improving patient care, particularly when associated with AS support. Local implementation of rapid methods, preparation of antibiograms, and interpretation of antimicrobial susceptibility tests should be done in partnership with pharmacy and clinicians versed in AS. This will ensure appropriate test use, a clear understanding of test characteristics and result interpretation, and opportunities for expert opinion to influence antimicrobial treatment.

DISCLOSURE

The authors have nothing to disclose.

REFERENCES

1. CDC. Antibiotic resistance threats in the United States, 2013. U.S. Department of Health and Human Services Centers for Disease Control and Prevention; 2013.
2. Shehab N, Patel PR, Srinivasan A, et al. Emergency department visits for antibiotic-associated adverse events. Clin Infect Dis 2008;47(6):735–43.
3. Ohl CA, Luther VP. Antimicrobial stewardship for inpatient facilities. J Hosp Med 2011;6(1):S4–15.
4. MacDougall C, Polk RE. Antimicrobial stewardship programs in health care systems. Clin Microbiol Rev 2005;18(4):638–56.
5. Dellit TH, Owens RC, McGowan JE Jr, et al. Infectious Diseases Society of America and the Society for Healthcare Epidemiology of America guidelines for developing an institutional program to enhance antimicrobial stewardship. Clin Infect Dis 2007;44(2):159–77.
6. Barlam TF, Cosgrove SE, Abbo LM, et al. Implementing an antibiotic stewardship program: guidelines by the Infectious Diseases Society of America and the Society for Healthcare Epidemiology of America. Clin Infect Dis 2016;62(10):e51–77.
7. CDC. Core elements of hospital antibiotic stewardship programs. Atlanta (GA): US Department of Health and Human Services, CDC; 2014.
8. The Joint Commission. Approved: new antimicrobial stewardship standard. Jt Comm Perspect 2016;36(7):1, 3–4,8.
9. CLSI. Performance standards for antimicrobial susceptibility testing. 29th edition. Wayne (PA): Clinical and Laboratory Standards Institute; 2019. CLSI supplement M100.
10. CLSI. Analysis and presentation of cumulative antimicrobial susceptibility test data, approved guideline—4th edition. CLSI document M39-A4. 4th edition. Wayne (PA): Clinical and Laboratory Standards Institute; 2014.
11. Beardsley JR, Williamson JC, Johnson JW, et al. Using local microbiologic data to develop institution-specific guidelines for the treatment of hospital-acquired pneumonia. Chest 2006;130(3):787–93.
12. Theel ES. Matrix-assisted laser desorption ionization-time of flight mass spectrometry for the identification of bacterial and fungal isolates. Clin Microbiol Newsl 2013;35(19):155–61.
13. Wieser A, Schneider L, Jung J, et al. MALDI-TOF MS in microbiological diagnostics-identification of microorganisms and beyond (mini review). Appl Microbiol Biotechnol 2012;93(3):965–74.
14. Levesque S, Dufresne PJ, Soualhine H, et al. A side by side comparison of Bruker Biotyper and VITEK MS: utility of MALDI-TOF MS technology for microorganism identification in a public health reference laboratory. PLoS One 2015;10(12): e0144878.
15. El-Bouri K, Johnston S, Rees E, et al. Comparison of bacterial identification by MALDI-TOF mass spectrometry and conventional diagnostic microbiology methods: agreement, speed and cost implications. Br J Biomed Sci 2012; 69(2):47–55.
16. Perez KK, Olsen RJ, Musick WL, et al. Integrating rapid pathogen identification and antimicrobial stewardship significantly decreases hospital costs. Arch Pathol Lab Med 2013;137(9):1247–54.
17. Huang AM, Newton D, Kunapuli A, et al. Impact of rapid organism identification via matrix-assisted laser desorption/ionization time-of-flight combined with antimicrobial stewardship team intervention in adult patients with bacteremia and candidemia. Clin Infect Dis 2013;57(9):1237–45.

18. Vlek AL, Bonten MJ, Boel CE. Direct matrix-assisted laser desorption ionization time-of-flight mass spectrometry improves appropriateness of antibiotic treatment of bacteremia. PLoS One 2012;7(3):e32589.

19. Lockwood AM, Perez KK, Musick WL, et al. Integrating rapid diagnostics and antimicrobial stewardship in two community hospitals improved process measures and antibiotic adjustment time. Infect Control Hosp Epidemiol 2016; 37(4):425–32.

20. Palavecino EL. Rapid methods for detection of MRSA in clinical specimens. In: Ji Y, editor. Methicillin-resistant *Staphylococcus aureus* (MRSA) protocols. Totowa (NJ): Humana Press; 2014. p. 71–83.

21. Harbarth S, Hawkey PM, Tenover F, et al. Update on screening and clinical diagnosis of methicillin-resistant *Staphylococcus aureus* (MRSA). Int J Antimicrob Agents 2011;37(2):110–7.

22. Palavecino E. One sample, multiple results: the use of multiplex PCR for diagnosis of infectious syndromes. Clin Laboratory News 2015.

23. Messacar K, Parker SK, Todd JK, et al. Implementation of rapid molecular infectious disease diagnostics: the role of diagnostic and antimicrobial stewardship. J Clin Microbiol 2017;55(3):715–23.

24. Kumar A, Ellis P, Arabi Y, et al. Initiation of inappropriate antimicrobial therapy results in a fivefold reduction of survival in human septic shock. Chest 2009;136(5): 1237–48.

25. Seymour CW, Gesten F, Prescott HC, et al. Time to treatment and mortality during mandated emergency care for sepsis. N Engl J Med 2017;376(23):2235–44.

26. Ward C, Stocker K, Begum J, et al. Performance evaluation of the Verigene (Nanosphere) and FilmArray (BioFire) molecular assays for identification of causative organisms in bacterial bloodstream infections. Eur J Clin Microbiol Infect Dis 2015;34(3):487–96.

27. Banerjee R, Teng CB, Cunningham SA, et al. Randomized trial of rapid multiplex polymerase chain reaction–based blood culture identification and susceptibility testing. Clin Infect Dis 2015;61(7):1071–80.

28. Neuner EA, Pallotta AM, Lam SW, et al. Experience with rapid microarray-based diagnostic technology and antimicrobial stewardship for patients with gram-positive bacteremia. Infect Control Hosp Epidemiol 2016;37(11):1361–6.

29. Wenzler E, Goff DA, Mangino JE, et al. Impact of rapid identification of *Acinetobacter baumannii* via matrix-assisted laser desorption ionization time-of-flight mass spectrometry combined with antimicrobial stewardship in patients with pneumonia and/or bacteremia. Diagn Microbiol Infect Dis 2016;84(1):63–8.

30. Bookstaver PB, Nimmich EB, Smith TJ 3rd, et al. Cumulative effect of an antimicrobial stewardship and rapid diagnostic testing bundle on early streamlining of antimicrobial therapy in gram-negative bloodstream infections. Antimicrob Agents Chemother 2017;61(9) [pii:e00189-17].

31. Timbrook TT, Morton JB, McConeghy KW, et al. The effect of molecular rapid diagnostic testing on clinical outcomes in bloodstream infections: a systematic review and meta-analysis. Clin Infect Dis 2016;64(1):15–23.

32. Schreckenberger PC, McAdam AJ. Point-counterpoint: large multiplex PCR panels should be first-line tests for detection of respiratory and intestinal pathogens. J Clin Microbiol 2015;53(10):3110–5.

33. Farthing M, Salam MA, Lindberg G, et al. Acute diarrhea in adults and children: a global perspective. J Clin Gastroenterol 2013;47(1):12–20.

34. Riddle MS, DuPont HL, Connor BA. ACG clinical guideline: diagnosis, treatment, and prevention of acute diarrheal infections in adults. Am J Gastroenterol 2016; 111(5):602–22.
35. Leber AL, Everhart K, Balada-Llasat JM, et al. Multicenter evaluation of Biofire FilmArray meningitis/encephalitis panel for detection of bacteria, viruses, and yeast in cerebrospinal fluid specimens. J Clin Microbiol 2016;54(9):2251–61.
36. Gomez CA, Pinsky BA, Liu A, et al. Delayed diagnosis of tuberculous meningitis misdiagnosed as herpes simplex virus-1 encephalitis with the FilmArray syndromic polymerase chain reaction panel. Open Forum Infect Dis 2017;4(1): ofw245.
37. Patel R, Fang FC. Diagnostic stewardship: opportunity for a laboratory-infectious diseases partnership. Clin Infect Dis 2018;67(5):799–801.
38. Morency-Potvin P, Schwartz DN, Weinstein RA. Antimicrobial stewardship: how the microbiology laboratory can right the ship. Clin Microbiol Rev 2017;30(1): 381–407.
39. Crobach MJ, Planche T, Eckert C, et al. European Society of Clinical Microbiology and Infectious Diseases: update of the diagnostic guidance document for *Clostridium difficile* infection. Clin Microbiol Infect 2016;22(Suppl 4):S63–81.
40. McDonald LC, Gerding DN, Johnson S, et al. Clinical practice guidelines for clostridium difficile infection in adults and children: 2017 update by the Infectious Diseases Society of America (IDSA) and Society for Healthcare Epidemiology of America (SHEA). Clin Infect Dis 2018;66(7):987–94.

Nurses and Antimicrobial Stewardship
Past, Present, and Future

Rita Drummond Olans, DNP, RN, CPNP-PC, APRN-BC[a],*,
Nicholas Bowditch Hausman, MBA[b], Richard Neal Olans, MD[c]

KEYWORDS

- Antimicrobial stewardship • Antimicrobial stewardship programs • Nurses
- Nursing communication • Nursing collaboration

KEY POINTS

- To be successful, antimicrobial stewardship must be a truly collaborative multidisciplinary team effort.
- Nurses have critical contributions to this effort and are starting to be recognized more in publications about antimicrobial stewardship.
- Examination of patient care workflow patterns indicates the central role of nurses in the application of antimicrobial stewardship concepts in the patient care setting.
- Education about antimicrobial resistance and antimicrobial stewardship is important not only for nurses and other health care providers but also for the general public.
- Analysis of the health care workforce population clearly shows the importance of integrating this largest segment of health care providers in the routine daily care of patients into all stewardship efforts.

Widespread resistance to antibiotics is an acknowledged national and global health crisis.[1] Although multifactorial in cause, inappropriate antibiotic use and overuse in health care settings is a major identified contributor to this problem.[2] The foremost strategy currently to address this increasing problem is antimicrobial stewardship (AS), the thoughtful and judicious use of antibiotics to achieve the best clinical outcome for individual patients while limiting the development and spread of multidrug-resistant microorganisms throughout society. AS success requires not only the awareness and education of both the public and health care workers about

[a] MGH Institute of Health Professions – School of Nursing, 36 First Avenue, Boston, MA 02129, USA; [b] MIT Sloan Office of External Relations, 100 Main Street, Cambridge, MA 02139, USA; [c] Melrose Wakefield Hospital, 585 Lebanon Street, Melrose, MA 02176, USA
* Corresponding author.
E-mail address: rolans@mghihp.edu

Infect Dis Clin N Am 34 (2020) 67–82
https://doi.org/10.1016/j.idc.2019.10.008
id.theclinics.com
0891-5520/20/© 2019 Elsevier Inc. All rights reserved.

this issue but also the training and collaboration of all health care providers to control this increasing threat to human health.

Antimicrobial stewardship programs (ASPs) and antibiotic use guidelines have been created in hospitals and nursing homes (NHs) to achieve these goals. These efforts have involved the Centers for Disease Control and Prevention (CDC), the Agency for Healthcare Research and Quality (AHRQ), hospitals, and health professional associations to address this serious problem. This article reviews the structure and function of ASPs with particular attention to the role of nurses in the stewardship process.

ANTIMICROBIAL STEWARDSHIP PROGRAMS AND NURSES: THE PAST

Formal ASPs have been developed only since the twenty-first century[3] and have included as stakeholders infectious diseases physicians, pharmacists, infection preventionists, and microbiologists, with support from administration and informatics.[4] Although guidelines for ASPs invariably highlight broad-based interdisciplinary involvement as critical for the successful achievement of AS goals, inclusion of frontline nursing is hardly mentioned.[5,6] The only nursing presence in early ASPs was infection control epidemiologists, often infection control nurses. Their contributions to AS efforts were largely the traditional surveillance, data gathering, and isolation functions, along with hospital-wide education on those topics for, among others, bedside nurses. Even after the White House[7] and CDC reports[8] on the scope and severity of the emerging dangers and costs of antibiotic resistant infections, scant mention was made of any nursing contributions to the stewardship process. The only published exceptions to this were 1 Australian and 1 British article that described bedside nursing activities that "should be implemented"[9] or "could impact"[10] antimicrobial stewardship efforts.

The first American paper to posit an important, integrated role of the bedside staff nurse in multiple stewardship activities was published in 2016.[11] The investigators asserted that many routine nursing functions were already critical components of existing ASP activities (**Table 1**). They conjectured that the failure of nursing to be included in ASP structures or planning could be due either (a) to a perception of infection preventionists as nurse representatives or (b) to the dearth of published articles on antibiotic resistance or antimicrobial stewardship in nursing journals.[12–14] There was also a perception among nurses themselves that, with the exception of nurse practitioners,[14] they were not antibiotic prescribers and therefore were not integral to AS functions.[15]

The CDC supported nursing inclusion in the National Quality Partners Playbook[16] in their core elements for antimicrobial stewardship. The CDC also collaborated with the American Nurses Association (ANA) in the development of a White Paper to redefine and clarify the roles of nurses in hospital antibiotic practices.[17] These documents were subsequently followed by The Joint Commission (TJC) Antimicrobial Stewardship Standard (MM.09.01.01),[18] requiring hospitals and nursing care centers to have multidisciplinary ASP teams. The Centers for Medicare and Medicaid Services (CMS) also put forward a requirement for participation rule requiring ASPs in long-term care facilities (LTCFs).[19]

NURSES AND ANTIMICROBIAL STEWARDSHIP: THE PRESENT

Fueled at least in part by the regulatory drive of TJC certification stewardship requirements and by CMS economic consequences, ASPs are increasing in number. Published articles on AS, including those that mention nurses, are also on the increase (**Figs. 1** and **2**). However, whereas those publications express optimism about nurse inclusion, most of the articles discuss theoretic constructs rather than describe

Table 1
Overlap of nursing activities with function attribution in current antimicrobial stewardship models

	Nursing	Microbiology	Case Management	Pharmacy	Infectious Diseases	Infection Preventionist	Hospitalist	Administration
Patient admission								
Triage and appropriate isolation	•					•		
Accurate allergy history	•			•	•		•	
Early and appropriate cultures	•	•			•		•	
Timely antibiotic initiation	•				•		•	•
Medication reconciliation	•			•			•	
Daily (24 h) clinical progress monitoring								
Progress monitor and report	•		•		•		•	
Preliminary micro results and antibiotic adjustment	•	•		•	•		•	
Antibiotic dosing and deescalation	•			•	•		•	
Patient safety & quality monitoring								
Adverse events	•			•	•		•	
Change in patient condition	•				•		•	

(continued on next page)

Table 1
(continued)

	Nursing	Microbiology	Case Management	Pharmacy	Infectious Diseases	Infection Preventionist	Hospitalist	Administration
Final culture report and antibiotic adjustment	•	•			•	•	•	
Antibiotic resistance identification	•	•			•	•	•	
Communication & patient education								
Device and antibiotic timeouts	•			•	•		•	
Interdisciplinary communication	•		•	•	•		•	•
Patient/family communication and education	•		•				•	
Clinical progress/discharge								
Intravenous to oral antibiotic, outpatient antibiotic therapy	•		•	•	•		•	
Medication reconciliation	•			•			•	
Length of stay	•		•		•		•	•
Outpatient management, long-term care, readmission	•		•		•	•		•

Adapted from Olans RN, Olans RD, Demaria, A Jr. The critical role of the staff nurse in antimicrobial stewardship–unrecognized, but already there. Clin Infect Dis 2016;62:84-9; with permission.

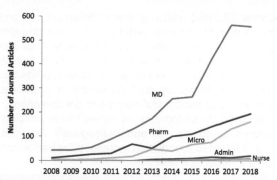

Fig. 1. Total number of AS publications by journal audience. Admin, Administration; MD, physician; Pharm, pharmacist; Micro, Microbiologist.

working models of nurse participation or evaluate operational nurse successes. Carter and colleagues[20] and Monsees and colleagues[21] surveyed nurses and identified nursing roles and barriers to nurse integration into ASPs. Olans and colleagues[22] and Monsees and colleagues[23] delineated specific activities already performed in daily practice by nurses that contribute to the AS paradigm while not being character- ized as such within currently existing ASPs. Surprisingly, however, Abbas and col- leagues[24] and Greendyke and colleagues[25] found that, despite those AS duties, between 35% and 62% of nurses were unfamiliar with the term antimicrobial steward- ship or were unaware that there was a functioning ASP in their own hospitals.

This raises the question: what *is* the nursing promise for antimicrobial stewardship programs and what evidence is there that it can work? Does this represent a negative publication bias (ie, that nurses are less likely to write up their successful accomplish- ments)? Or is it that collaborative interprofessional nursing/medical endeavors are either rare or rarely successful? In a review by Martin and colleagues[26] of 14 randomly controlled trials of interprofessional collaboration among physicians and nurses, at least 1 statistically significant improvement in patient outcomes was found in 13 of the 14 studies. However, in a 3-part series of articles on teamwork challenges pub- lished in the *New England Journal of Medicine*,[27–29] the word "nurse" appears only 4 times, none of which are in the context of teamwork functions.

In the realm of antimicrobial stewardship and infection prevention, one of the most dramatic teamwork success stories has been the reduction of central line-associated

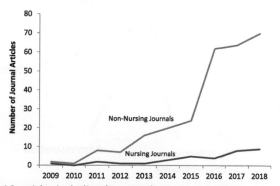

Fig. 2. Published AS articles including key words nurse or nursing.

bloodstream infections (CLABSI) following the involvement of frontline nurses in a CLABSI bundle intervention.[30] Likewise, regular staff nurse prompting and removal of urinary catheters were shown to reduce both the number of indwelling catheter days and the number of catheter-associated urinary tract infections (CAUTIs).[31] Although both CLABSIs and CAUTIs were initially identified as infection control issues, their operation was accomplished by staff nurse-driven protocols. Despite these large-scale demonstrations of successful nurse-led collaborations, the authors are aware of only a single report of incorporation of nurses into an existing ASP with resulting improved measured outcomes. Ha and colleagues[32] describe a nurse-driven model of stewardship-integrated rounds that increased the performance of a preexisting acute care audit-and-feedback ASP.

Allowing for the fact that nurses "touch" almost everything involved in antimicrobial stewardship, what additional factors/skills do nurses bring to the stewardship table? If one maps the daily workflow of the staff nurse and of ASP participants, the overlap becomes obvious (see **Table 1**). The bedside nurse is at the hub of a circumferential stewardship wheel (**Fig. 3**). This functional reality requires her/him to be the navigator of the numerous diagnostic and therapeutic tests associated with a patient's care. She/he is also the recipient of that patient's results and must prioritize and accurately communicate that data to all of the patient's caregivers.

All of this takes place coincident with the nurse's primary responsibilities of monitoring patients' clinical status and protecting patient safety. These duties require not only broad-based nurse education but also diverse communication skills to update all of the AS stakeholders as well as to inform the patient and the patient's family. Methods of communication (**Box 1**) are emphasized throughout prelicensure nursing education and can regularly provide interdisciplinary lubrication as well as the not uncommon discovery of a nugget of diagnostic significance. Nurse comfort with this communication[33] is even more important in an era when the benefit of a multidisciplinary stewardship culture is operationally evolving.[23,34]

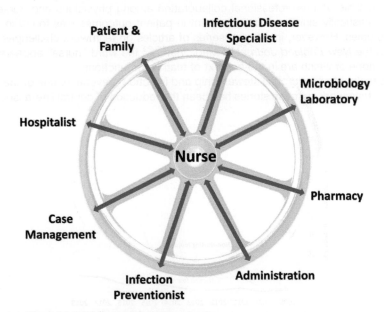

Fig. 3. Inpatient AS workflow and communications.

> **Box 1**
> **Examples of nurse communication techniques taught in nursing school and used in practice**
>
> Allowing silences to invite reflection and questions
>
> Appropriate touch
>
> Hi-fidelity and lo-fidelity simulation
>
> Identification of Maslow's Hierarchy of Needs and honoring the patient's circumstance
>
> Identify patient's register of language & speak in a vocabulary that is of comfort to the patient
>
> Motivational interviewing
>
> Observation of and use of body language
>
> Peer-2-Peer, Think-Pair-Share, Muddle Questions
>
> Reflection
>
> Role-playing
>
> SBAR (Situation, Background, Assessment, Recommendation)
>
> SBIRT (Screening, Brief Intervention, Referral to Treatment)
>
> Sensitive communication within patient's cultural understandings and beliefs
>
> Teach-back

At a time when optimal shorter durations of antibiotic therapy are being determined by individual patient response rather than by convenient multiples of 5 or 7 days, regular input from the bedside nurse becomes even more important in guiding appropriate treatment.[35] As laboratory results "chase" the patient to his or her bedside, the bedside nurse's communications to the prescribers not only have the safety imperatives of timing and reporting accuracy but also are linked with any nurse-guided stewardship nudges that a health care institution uses.[36,37] Examples of such AS interventions include the timing of specimen collection for appropriate *Clostridioides difficile* infection,[38] or Foley catheter discontinuation for CAUTI prevention.[39] Compliance with these guidelines is often more successful by persuasion than by fiat.[37,40]

Publications demonstrating the value of nurses in antimicrobial stewardship are most common in the setting of NHs and LTCFs. Morrill and colleagues[36] reviewed the interventions that have been implemented along with several other roles for nurses in the improvement of antimicrobial use in LTCFs. Scales and colleagues[41] surveyed the perspectives of nurses and physicians about AS in NHs and identified the nurse perception of the influence of patient families on antibiotic prescribing decisions.[41] Heath and colleagues[42] and Jump and colleagues[43] identified the need for education of nurses at many levels for the treatment of infections in older adults. Katz and colleagues[44] reviewed the literature on successful interventions in LTCFs and noted that multidisciplinary education and tools integrated into the workflow of nurses and of antibiotic prescribers reduced the number of unnecessary urine cultures 2-fold. Witts and Patterson[45] also reported success in decreasing asymptomatic bacteriuria overtreatment. Zabarsky and colleagues[46] successfully used such educational efforts to reduce total antibiotic use by 30%, maintained over the study period of 30 months. Trautner and colleagues[47] achieved similar decreases in urine culture ordering and in overtreatment of asymptomatic bacteriuria with a multifaceted education and guidelines intervention.

As described in the reports above, the education of nurses about antimicrobial resistance and nurses' contributions to AS is a recurring theme. In the latest position paper from Association for Professionals in Infection Control and Epidemiology/Society for Healthcare Epidemiology of America (SHEA)/Society of Infectious Diseases Pharmacists,[48] the importance of antimicrobial resistance (AMR) and AS education to all health care providers, including nurses, is also highlighted. AS information applications for nurses[49] and online courses to improve nurses' awareness of their role in AS[42,50] have also been described. Such efforts can begin to fill the identified gap in practicing nurses' education about antibiotic use,[51] antimicrobial resistance,[13] and antimicrobial stewardship.[14] In the United Kingdom, such education begins in nursing school[52] and is regarded as a central tenet for the establishment of national AS competencies.[53]

The most comprehensive approach to broad-based education about AMR and AS exists in the United Kingdom,[54] where AS educational programs teach appropriate antibiotic use to all health care professionals, including nurses, physicians, pharmacists, dentists, and veterinarians. Likewise, the Scottish Antimicrobial Prescribing Group[55] has produced extensive multimedia and multidisciplinary training materials for undergraduate as well as for postgraduate education. Such a broad-based, one-world educational approach brings nurses into the stewardship educational efforts to address spreading antimicrobial resistance.

As for the current status of AS nursing education in the United States, analysis of the English language publications on AS and AMR is revealing (see **Figs. 1** and **2**). Sym and colleagues[51] and Manning and colleagues[48] have pointed out the lack of formal AS education designed for nursing. Review of the last 10 years of publications on AS and AMR reveals an asymmetrical distribution of publications with medical (ie, infectious diseases and infection control) and pharmacy journals clearly dwarfing their nursing journal counterparts when it comes to numbers of publications. **Fig. 2** indicates that most AS literature is not published in nursing journals. Even when nurses are involved as authors, or cited, their work is overwhelmingly found in nonnursing journals.

This publication siloing unfortunately mirrors the past history of stewardship program organization; nursing involvement in AS efforts is viewed more frequently as infection control or prevention topics (eg, *American Journal of Infection Control* and *Infection Control and Hospital Epidemiology*) rather than being seen in the realm of daily nursing practice. Nonetheless, awareness of nursing AS relevance is increasing. As recognized in the National Quality Forum (NQF) playbook[16] and the ANA/CDC White Paper.[17] National stewardship planning efforts by the AHRQ continue to recognize the important role of nurses in the acute, long-term, and ambulatory settings. Their initiatives will clearly emphasize that it is time to bring nurses into stewardship practice. Through a variety of venues, the role of nurses in stewardship is being emphasized.

NURSES AND ANTIMICROBIAL STEWARDSHIP: THE FUTURE

Although antimicrobial stewardship programs had been in place in several hospitals since the turn of this century, the widespread use of the term antimicrobial stewardship[4] dates to 2007 with the publications of the first Infectious Diseases Society of America/Society for Healthcare Epidemiology of America Guidelines[5] for such programs. That document stated that ASPs should be multidisciplinary but did not specifically identify any roles for frontline staff nurses. Nurse inclusion was first widely publicized in the NQF Playbook[16] and by a *Clinical Infectious Diseases* publication in 2016.[11] Since that time, widespread institutionalization of ASPs and consideration of staff nurse stewardship participation have stimulated a spike in papers linking nursing with stewardship.

Despite this literary proliferation, those articles have largely been limited to analyses of *potential* nurse contributions rather than reporting results of *actual* nursing performance. Apart from the CLABSI and CAUTI success stories, the authors are aware of only a single report to of the development of a nurse-included ASP in acute care with measurements of its outcomes. Ha and colleagues[32] created a program of nurse-driven stewardship and infection control rounds in a community hospital with a preexisting hospital-wide conventional ASP with functional audit-and-feedback in place. With support from the hospital administration and board, Ha trained 2 nurse leaders/champions in AS basic precepts. The pharmacist and the unit nursing staff conducted twice weekly nurse-driven AS rounds. Those rounds generated stewardship recommendations communicated back to the prescribing physicians by the individual bedside staff nurses. Complex treatment issues or discordant treatment choices with the prescribing physicians were referred to the traditional infectious diseases physician-led ASP.

As the AS/infectious diseases pharmacist, Ha bridged communication between the parallel ASPs. Over 1 year, the nursing intervention was associated with a decrease of total antibiotic use and specifically of broad-spectrum antibiotics for treatment of community-acquired pneumonia. There were also decreases in central venous catheter and bladder catheter days as well as proton pump inhibitor use, unit length of stay, and hospital-onset *C difficile* infections.

The study demonstrated several additional surprising operational benefits. Tangible support was obtained from the hospital board and administration to enable the inception of the project. The leadership and empowerment of a respected nurse team leader and champion provided credibility and reassurance to the nursing staff that they were not having an additional task foisted upon them. Ha either showed or convinced them that they were working better, not harder. Positive feedback spread from the initial test site to nursing staff in other units. They viewed the bidirectional AS communication as improved nursing care rather than as a regulatory imposition. Additional units asked to be included in the stewardship initiative as well. Their enthusiasm promoted a broader awareness and increased consultations for the existing medical ASP.[32] The success engendered by administration endorsement and respected nurse stewardship champions conforms to key core elements of successful ASPs.[56]

Contrast this experience with that of Abbas and colleagues[24] at an 850-bed tertiary academic center with a 20-year-old established ASP. On surveying their more than 3000-person nursing staff, they discovered that 25% of the nurses did not know that the ASP existed and 80% had never communicated with the stewardship program. Such a description must be viewed not simply as a report of a curious dichotomy but as documentation of a stewardship failure. The authors acknowledged that nurse engagement in AS presents great opportunities for ASPs. The program is now embarking on an educational outreach to their nursing staff. Such collaboration could be beneficial for both the nurses and the ASP in a cooperative workplace. Even at a hospital with an established ASP, the integration of nurses can have beneficial results. In an evolving era of shortening durations of antibiotic therapy,[35] the daily input of the bedside nurse with stewardship communication (see **Fig. 3**) can be even more valuable. Both the ASP and the nurses could realize gains by recognizing each other's strengths. Each discipline's performance could improve by appreciating that: *"good nursing is good antimicrobial stewardship, and good antimicrobial stewardship is good nursing."*[22]

However, being multidisciplinary is not the same as being multicollaborative. To reverse the current trend of antibiotic overuse will require cooperation, communication, and education. ASPs need to appreciate and use all contributors to that end. Solving the antibiotic resistance crisis is everyone's goal. Only by recognizing and better understanding each discipline's roles and contributions to AS can we together create a safer, more collaborative, and better integrated stewardship process. Achieving this can improve individual patient as well as broader public health, now and in the future.

The CDC,[8] the World Health Organization,[57] and the World Economic Forum[58] predict ever more frightening numbers of lives and dollars lost to the ravages of drug-resistant infections. In this twenty-first century world of expanding antimicrobial resistance, when it can be difficult to quantify the progress of ASPs,[59] numbers of AS advocates is 1 measure of stewardship success or failure. Numbers also measure the members of the US health care workforce: 7000 infection preventionists,[60] 9100 infectious diseases physicians,[61] 700 board-certified infectious disease pharmacists,[62] 309,000 pharmacists,[63] 940,000 actively practicing physicians,[64] and 3.9 million nurses.[65]

Nurses are ubiquitous throughout the health care system and society. They practice within identified AS settings, such as hospitals, long-term care and skilled nursing facilities, and ambulatory care. However, nurses also practice in public health, schools, hospices, and nontraditional health care settings (**Box 2**). They deliver immunizations, teach health in classrooms, bring care into the home, and complement care delivered in community practices. Nurses practice in settings where stewardship efforts are

---

Box 2
Traditional and nontraditional settings for nursing antimicrobial stewardship

Acute care hospitals

Community health centers

Dialysis centers

Government and regulatory agencies

Homecare services and visiting nurses associations

Hospices

Industry

Insurance companies

Long-term care facilities

Military

Occupational health

Outpatient clinics

Physicians' offices

Prisons

Public health

Rehabilitation hospitals

Schools

Urgent care clinics

already underway and could provide a bridge into settings where stewardship needs to become more active. Antimicrobial resistance is a problem in all of these sites. Nurses will need to learn how best to apply the principles of AS to their competencies in each of these settings, because it is well documented how antibiotic-resistant pathogens can disseminate broadly throughout various health care facilities.[66,67]

In the annual US Gallup poll[68] of the public's trust in professions, nurses have been at the top of the list for 17 of the last 18 years. In this time of national and global crises of antibiotic resistance, we cannot neglect the potential impact of this largest group of health care professionals. Nurses are the most numerous and most trusted group of health care workers in society.[68] It only makes sense to include them in the critical efforts to limit the spread of antibiotic resistance. They cannot be left uninformed about the new realities of how best to use these valuable antibiotics.[69] Nurses must become active participants in stewardship activities as well as collaborative partners in community and public education about the prudent use of antimicrobials for human health in the twenty-first century.[70–72]

The CDC core measures of antimicrobial stewardship recognize the importance of respected leaders not only in hospital ASPs but also for the entire AS effort. Great leaders need good followers, as many of them as possible. Without his army, Alexander the Great might be remembered as Alexander the Merely Adequate. Just as to win a battle, one needs soldiers; to win a campaign, one needs supporters. To create a culture of change such as antimicrobial stewardship, one needs a large force of well-informed, credible, and committed participants. The leaders of ASPs, whether infectious disease physicians or pharmacists, need to recognize that numerical reality.[73,74]

The time has passed to continue writing papers about how nurses "could" or "might" become involved in stewardship. It is time to move beyond promoting nurse inclusion as a useful theoretic proposition and to work on applied interdisciplinary research to evaluate the actual optimal methods to achieve maximum patient- and society-based outcomes. The question is not *whether* or *when* nurses should be included, but rather how can the goals and outcomes of AS be adequately and maximally accomplished without recruiting the largest segment of the health care workforce, nurses (**Fig. 4**). The time has come to research the most productive working models of AS that incorporate nurses in all settings: acute care, NHs, LTCFs, as

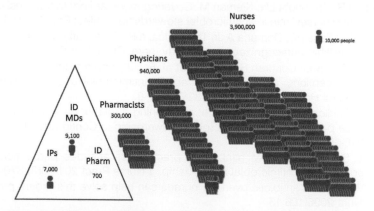

Fig. 4. Health care workforce numbers. Traditional Antimicrobial Stewardship Program participants in triangle. ID MDs, Infectious Disease Physicians; ID Pharm, Infectious Disease Pharmacists; IPs, infection preventionists.

well as outpatient and community/public health. AS has always been described as, and must function as, a collaborative team effort. We can all be antimicrobial stewards together or we can remain (multi)resistant apart.

DISCLOSURE

The authors have nothing to disclose.

REFERENCES

1. Bartlett JG. A call to arms: the imperative for antimicrobial stewardship. Clin Infect Dis 2011;53(s1):s4–7.
2. Fridkin S, Baggs J, Fagan R, et al. Vital signs: improving antibiotic use among hospitalized patients. MMWR Morb Mortal Wkly Rep 2014;63(9):194–200.
3. Gross R, Morgan AS, Kinky DE, et al. Impact of a hospital-based antimicrobial program on clinical and economic outcomes. Clin Infect Dis 2001;33:289–95.
4. Fishman N. Antimicrobial stewardship. Am J Med 2006;119(suppl 1):S53–61.
5. Dellit TH, Owens RC, McGowan JE Jr. Infectious Diseases Society of America and the Society for Healthcare Epidemiology of America guidelines for developing an institutional program to enhance antimicrobial stewardship. Clin Infect Dis 2007;44:159–77.
6. American Society of Health System Pharmacists. An interprofessional approach to antimicrobial stewardship: implementing team-based strategies that impact patient outcomes. Available at: http://www.leadstewardship.org. Accessed December 29, 2014.
7. The White House. National action plan for combating antibiotic-resistant bacteria. 2015. Available at: https://obamawhitehouse.archives.gov/sites/default/files/docs/national_action_plan_for_combating_antibotic-resistant_bacteria.pdf. Accessed March 31, 2019.
8. Centers for Disease Control and Prevention. Antibiotic resistance threats in the United States, 2013. 2013. Atlanta. Available at: https://www.cdc.gov/drugresistance/pdf/ar-threats-2013-508.pdf. Accessed March 23, 2019.
9. Gillespie E, Rodrigues A, Wright L, et al. Improving antibiotic stewardship by involving nurses. Am J Infect Control 2013;41:365–7.
10. Edwards R, Drumright LN, Kieman M. Covering more territory to fight resistance: considering nurses' role in antimicrobial stewardship. J Infect Prev 2011;12:6–10.
11. Olans RN, Olans RD, Demaria A Jr. The critical role of the staff nurse in antimicrobial stewardship-unrecognized, but already there. Clin Infect Dis 2016;62:84–9.
12. Abbo L, Sinkowitz-Cochran R, Smith L, et al. Faculty and resident physicians' attitudes, perceptions, and knowledge about antimicrobial use and resistance. Infect Control Hosp Epidemiol 2011;32(7):714–8.
13. Olans RD, Nicholas PK, Hanley D, et al. Defining a role for nursing education in staff nurse participation in antimicrobial stewardship. J Contin Educ Nurs 2015; 46(7):318–21.
14. Abbo L, Smith L, Pereyra M, et al. Nurse practitioners' attitudes, perceptions, and knowledge about antimicrobial stewardship. J Nurse Pract 2012;8(5):370–6.
15. Hart AM. Against antibiotic overuse: nurses can help solve this urgent problem. Am J Nurs 2006;106:13.
16. National Quality Partners Playbook: antibiotic stewardship in acute care playbook. 2016. Available at: https://www.qualityforum.org/aqp/antibiotic_stewardship_playbook.aspx. Accessed March 19, 2019.

17. ANA/CDC White Paper. Redefining the antibiotic stewardship team: recommendations from the American Nurses Association/Centers for Disease Control and Prevention workgroup on the role of registered nurses in hospital antibiotic stewardship practices. Available at: https://www.cdc.gov/antibiotic-use/healthcare/pdfs/ANA-CDC-whitepaper.pdf. Accessed March 20,2019.
18. The Joint Commission (TJC) Antimicrobial Stewardship Standard (MM.09.01.01) 2017. Available at: https://www.jointcommission.org/assets/.../New_Antimicrobial_Stewardship_Standard.pdf. Accessed March 21, 2019.
19. Centers for Medicare and Medicaid Services-CMS.gov. Section 1.C. Systems to prevent transmission of MDROs and promote antimicrobial stewardship. Available at: https://www.cms.gov/medicare...and.../survey-and-cert-letter-15-12-attachment-1.pdf. Accessed March 19, 2019.
20. Carter EJ, Greendyke WG, Furuya EY, et al. Exploring the nurses' role in antibiotic stewardship: a multisite qualitative study of nurses and infection preventionists. Am J Infect Control 2018;46:492–7.
21. Monsees E, Popejoy L, Jackson MA, et al. Integrating staff nurses in antibiotic stewardship: opportunities and barriers. Am J Infect Control 2018;46:737–42.
22. Olans RD, Olans RN, Witt DJ. Good nursing is good antibiotic stewardship. Am J Nurs 2017;117(8):58–63.
23. Monsees E, Tamma P, Cosgrove SE. Integrating bedside nurses into antibiotic stewardship: a practical approach. Infect Control Hosp Epidemiol 2019;40(5):579–84.
24. Abbas S, Lee K, Pakcyz A, et al. Knowledge, attitudes and practices of bedside nursing staff regarding antibiotic stewardship: a cross-sectional study. Am J Infect Control 2019;47(3):230–3.
25. Greendyke W, Carter EJ, Salsgiver E, et al. Clinical nurses are active partners in antimicrobials stewardship efforts: results from a multisite survey. Open Forum Infect Dis 2016;3(1):965.
26. Martin JS, Ummenhofer W, Manser T, et al. Interprofessional collaboration among nurses and physicians: making a difference in patient outcome. Swiss Med Wkly 2010;140:w13062.
27. Rosenbaum L. Medicine and Society. Teamwork - Part 1. Divided we fall. N Engl J Med 2019;380(7):684–8.
28. Rosenbaum L. Medicine and Society. Teamwork-Part 2. Cursed by knowledge-building a culture of psychological safety. N Engl J Med 2019;380(7):786–90.
29. Rosenbaum L. Medicine and Society. Teamwork-Part 3. The not-my-problem problem. N Engl J Med 2019;380(7):881–5.
30. Furuya EY, Dick A, Prencevich EN. Central line bundle implementation in US intensive care units and impact on bloodstream infections. PLoS One 2011;6(1):e15452.
31. Saint S, Greene T, Krein S, et al. A program to prevent catheter-associated urinary tract infection in acute care. N Engl J Med 2016;374(22):2111–9.
32. Ha D, Forte MB, Olans R, et al. A multi-disciplinary approach to incorporate bedside nurses into antimicrobial stewardship and infection prevention. Jt Comm J Qual Patient Saf 2019. https://doi.org/10.1016/jcjq.2019.03.003.
33. Apker J, Propp KM, Zabava Ford WS, et al. Collaboration, credibility, compassion, and coordination: professional nurse communication skill sets in healthcare team interactions. J Prof Nurs 2006;22(3):180–9.
34. Charani E, Castro-Sanchez E, Holmes A. The role of behavior change in antimicrobial stewardship. Infect Dis Clin North Am 2014;28(2):169–75.

35. Spellberg B. The new antibiotic mantra-"shorter is better". In JAMA Intern Med. 2016. Available at: https://www.ncbi.nlm.nih.gov/pmc/articles/PMC5233409/. Accessed March 22, 2019.

36. Morrill HJ, Caffrey AR, Jump RLP, et al. Antimicrobial stewardship in long-term care facilities: a call to action. J Am Med Dir Assoc 2016;17(2):183e1–16.

37. Spellberg B. Antibiotic judo: working gently with prescriber psychology to overcome inappropriate use. JAMA Intern Med 2014;174(3):432–3.

38. Bruno-Murtha LA, Osgood RA, Alexandre CE. A successful strategy to decrease hospital-onset Clostridium difficile. Infect Control Hosp Epidemiol 2018;39(2): 234–6.

39. Parry MF, Grant B, Sestovic M. Successful reduction in catheter-associated urinary tract infections: focus on nurse-directed catheter removal. Am J Infect Control 2013;41(12):1178–81.

40. Goldstein EJC, Goff DA, Reeve W, et al. Approaches to modifying the behavior of clinicians who are noncompliant with antimicrobial stewardship program guidelines. Clin Infect Dis 2016;63(4):532–8.

41. Scales K, Zimmerman S, Reed D, et al. Nurse and medical provider perspectives on antibiotic stewardship in nursing homes. J Am Geriatr Soc 2017;65(1):165–71.

42. Heath B, Bernhardt J, Michalski TJ, et al. Results of a Veterans Affairs employee education program on antimicrobial stewardship for older adults. Am J Infect Control 2016;44(3):349–51.

43. Jump RL, Heath B, Crnich CJ, et al. Knowledge, beliefs, and confidence regarding infections and antimicrobial stewardship: a survey of Veterans Affairs providers who care for older adults. Am J Infect Control 2015;43(3):298–300.

44. Katz MJ, Gurses AP, Tamma PD, et al. Implementing antimicrobial stewardship in long-term care settings: an integrative review using a human factors approach. Clin Infect Dis 2017;65(11):1943–51.

45. Witts KD, Patterson PP. Antibiotic stewardship: the nurses' role in making a difference. Am J Infect Control 2016;44:s28.

46. Zabarsky TF, Sethi AK, Donskey CJ. Sustained reduction in inappropriate treatment of asymptomatic bacteriuria in a long-term care facility through an educational intervention. Am J Infect Control 2008;36:476–80.

47. Trautner BW, Grigoryan L, Petersen NJ, et al. Effectiveness of an antimicrobial stewardship approach for urinary catheter-asymptomatic bacteriuria. JAMA Intern Med 2015;175(7):1120–7.

48. Manning ML, Septimius EJ, Dodds Ashley E, et al. APIC/SHEA/SIDP Antimicrobial Stewardship Position Paper. Antimicrobial stewardship and infection prevention-leveraging the synergy: a position paper update. Am J Infect Control 2018;46: 364–8.

49. Wentzel J, van Drie-Pierik R, Nijdam L, et al. Antibiotic information application offers nurses quick support. Am J Infect Control 2016;44(6):677–84.

50. Wilson BM, Shick S, Carter RR, et al. An online course improves nurses' awareness of their role as antimicrobial stewards in nursing homes. Am J Infect Control 2017;45(5):466–70.

51. Sym D, Brennan CW, Hart AM, et al. Characteristics of nurse practitioner curricular in the United States related to antimicrobial prescribing and resistance. J Am Acad Nurse Pract 2007;19(9):477–85.

52. McEwen J, Burnett E. Antimicrobial stewardship and pre-registration student nurses: evaluation of teaching. J Infect Prev 2018;19:80–6.

53. Courtenay M, Lim R, Castro-Sanchez E, et al. Development of consensus-based national antimicrobial stewardship competencies for UK undergraduate healthcare professional education. J Hosp Infect 2018;100(3):245–56.
54. Castro-Sanchez E, Drumright LN, Gharbi M, et al. Mapping antimicrobial stewardship in undergraduate medical, dental, pharmacy, nursing and veterinary education in the United Kingdom. PLoS One 2016;11(2):e0150056. Available at: https://www.ncbi.nlm.nih.gov/pubmed/26928009.
55. Scottish Antimicrobial Prescribing Group [SAPG]. Education. Available at: https://www.sapg.scot/education/. Accessed March 31, 2019.
56. Goff DA, Kullar R, Bauer KA, et al. Eight habits of highly effective antimicrobial stewardship programs to meet the Joint Commission standards for hospitals. Clin Infect Dis 2017;64:1134–9.
57. World Health Organization (WHO). High levels of antibiotic resistance found worldwide, new data shows. 2019. Available at: https://www.who.int/news-room/detail/29-01-2018-high-levels-of-antibiotic-resistance-found-worldwide-new-data-shows. Accessed March 31, 2019.
58. World Economic Forum. Antimicrobial resistance. 2018. Available at: http://reports.weforum.org/global-risks-2018/anti-microbial-resistance/. Accessed March 20, 2019.
59. Dodds-Ashely ES, Kaye KS, DePestel DD, et al. Antimicrobial stewardship: philosophy versus practice. Clin Infect Dis 2014;59(suppl 3):S112–21.
60. Certification Board of Infection Control and Epidemiology. CIC fast facts. Available at: https://www.cbic.org/CBIC.htm. Accessed March 20, 2019.
61. Statista. The statistics portal. Available at: https://www.statista.com/statistics/439728/active-physicians-by-specialty-and-gender-in-the-us/. Accessed March 18, 2019.
62. Board of Pharmacy Specialties. Infectious disease specialists. Available at: https://portalbps.cyzap.net/dzapps/dbzap.bin/apps/assess/webmembers/managetool?webid=BPS&pToolCode=certrecord&pRecCmd=StatsByLocation&pPrint=Yes&pLandScape=Yes. Accessed June 9, 2019.
63. United States Department of Labor: Bureau of Labor Statistics. Occupational employment statistics. Occupational employment and wages, May 2017. Pharmacists. 2018. Available at: https://www.bls.gov/oes/2017/may/oes291051.htm. Accessed March 20, 2019.
64. Statista. U.S. Physicians–Statistics & facts. Available at: https://www.statista.com/topics/1244/physicians/. Accessed March 18, 2019.
65. Haddad LM, Toney-Butler TJ. Nursing shortage. StatPearls. Available at: https://www.ncbi.nlm.nih.gov/books/NBK493175/. Accessed March 18, 2019.
66. Datta R, Brown S, Nguyen VQ, et al. Quantifying the exposure to antibiotic-resistant pathogens among patients discharged from a single hospital across all California healthcare facilities. Infect Control Hosp Epidemiol 2015;36(11):1275–82.
67. Jump RLP, Gaur S, Katz MJ, et al. Infection advisory committee for AMDA–the Society for Post-Acute and Long-Term Care Medicine. Template for an antibiotic stewardship policy for post-acute and long-term care settings. J Am Med Dir Assoc 2017;18(11):913–20.
68. Gallup. Nurses again outpace other professions for honesty, ethics. 2018. Available at: https://news.gallup.com/poll/245597/nurses-again-outpace-professions-honesty-ethics.aspx. Accessed March 31, 2019.
69. Spellberg B. New societal approaches to empowering antibiotic stewardship. JAMA 2016;315(12):1229–30.

70. Castro-Sanchez E. European Commission guidelines for the prudent use of anti-microbials in human health: a missed opportunity to embrace nursing participation in stewardship. Clin Microbiol Infect 2018;24:914–5.
71. Pulcini C, Morel CM, Tacconelli E, et al. Human resources estimates and funding for antibiotic stewardship team are urgently needed. Clin Microbiol Infect 2017; 23:785–7.
72. Wiley KC, Villamizar HJ. Antibiotic resistance policy and the stewardship role of the nurse. Policy Polit Nurs Pract 2019;20(1):8–17.
73. Ostrovsky B, Banerjee R, Bonomo R, et al. Infectious diseases physicians: leading the way in antimicrobial stewardship. Clin Infect Dis 2018;66:995–1003.
74. Dodds-Ashley E, Davis SL, Heil EL, et al. Best care for patients achieved through multidisciplinary stewardship. Clin Infect Dis 2018;67(10):1637.

Stewardship-Hospitalist Collaboration

Megan Mack, MD[a], Adamo Brancaccio, PharmD[b], Kayla Popova, PharmD[b], Jerod Nagel, PharmD[b],*

KEYWORDS

- Antibiotic stewardship • Antimicrobial stewardship • Hospitalist • Collaboration

KEY POINTS

- Hospitalists represent the fasted growing subspecialty, which provides care to the majority of hospitalized patients with community-acquired infections, and represents an ideal target group for stewardship collaboration.
- Numerous Hospitalist-Stewardship studies demonstrate that collaborative interventions can improve antimicrobial prescribing and clinical outcomes.
- Utilizing a multifaceted collaborative model can help optimize implementation of Hospitalist-Stewardship initiatives and avoid potential barriers to success.

INTRODUCTION

Hospitalists are the fastest growing group of specialty practitioners in the United States.[1] At many major academic medical centers, hospitalists represent the largest division of physicians treating adult patients, and there is a similar and emerging trend among hospitalists treating pediatric patients.[2] Adult and pediatric hospitalists treat a large percentage of patients admitted for the management of infections.[3] Hospitalists are in a prime position to execute antimicrobial stewardship practices for multiple reasons, including their frontline provider perspective, the growing number of hospitalists compared with infectious disease specialists, as well as the type and quantity of antimicrobials they prescribe.[4–6] Thus, building a collaborative stewardship and hospitalist partnership provides the opportunity to improve antimicrobial stewardship and affect patient outcomes. In addition, hospitalists frequently provide mentorship to medical interns and residents and have significant influence on antimicrobial stewardship knowledge, attitudes, and skills of young trainees.[3]

Hospitalists are positioned to play an active role in antimicrobial stewardship programs in a variety of ways.[7–10] They can directly affect antimicrobial stewardship by

[a] Department of Internal Medicine, Michigan Medicine, University of Michigan, School of Medicine, 1500 East Medical Center Drive, Ann Arbor, MI 48109, USA; [b] Department of Pharmacy Services, Michigan Medicine, University of Michigan, College of Pharmacy, 1500 East Medical Center Drive, Ann Arbor, MI 48109, USA
* Corresponding author.
E-mail address: nageljl@umich.edu

Infect Dis Clin N Am 34 (2020) 83–96
https://doi.org/10.1016/j.idc.2019.11.001
0891-5520/20/© 2019 Elsevier Inc. All rights reserved.

id.theclinics.com

selecting appropriate empiric antimicrobial therapy, providing prompt de-escalation of antimicrobial agents and ensuring a correct duration of treatment, as well as adherence with performance measures for specific diseases.[7,10] By using frontline health care providers, antimicrobial stewardship teams can expand their impact on antimicrobial prescribing.[11]

There are many reasons for hospitalists to collaborate with stewardship programs, and vice versa. Antimicrobial stewardship programs have successfully demonstrated the ability to reduce unnecessary antimicrobial exposure, which often requires collaboration with various groups within the hospital to implement initiatives and affect patient outcomes.[12] Antimicrobial stewardship teams have the expertise, resources, and experience in helping to identify and implement change that affects antimicrobial prescribing. In addition, implementation of an antimicrobial stewardship program is required for accreditation by The Joint Commission when surveying acute care hospitals, long-term care facilities, and ambulatory clinics within a health care system, and hospitalists are likely to get involved in stewardship efforts as a hospital priority.[13] The Center of Medicare and Medicaid Services (CMS) set infection-related benchmarks that impact hospital reimbursement, and benchmarks are directly or indirectly affected by antimicrobial stewardship efforts.

Developing a hospitalist-antimicrobial stewardship collaboration should be based on tools and experiences demonstrated to be successful. The importance of developing a shared vision, trust, and assigned responsibilities, in addition to open communication, is imperative for optimizing outcomes. This review focuses on the unique approach, tools, and challenges in building successful antimicrobial stewardship-hospitalist collaboration.

USING A COLLABORATIVE MODEL TO IMPROVE STEWARDSHIP-HOSPITALIST EFFORTS

Building effective collaborations among health care providers is well documented in the literature and should use mechanisms and tools that have demonstrated success.[14] Setting the foundation for successful collaboration is just as important as picking a specific stewardship target or metric and requires joint planning, mutual discussion, and agreement.

D'Amour and colleagues[15] describe a model for collaboration of professionals within a health care system that could be the framework for antimicrobial stewardship and hospitalist collaboration. They describe a model with 4 primary pillars, and 10 indicators of collaboration associated with those primary pillars (**Table 1**). The 4 primary pillars include: Shared vision and goals; Governance; Formalization; and Internalization. Many of the key components of the D'Amour model are essential for successful antimicrobial stewardship and hospitalist collaboration. Establishing good coleadership, which agrees on common goals and develops a plan for implementation, is essential. Equally important is the ability to "focus on the details" when building a collaborative relationship. Each party must provide frequent and honest communication; understand the responsibilities of each party; develop necessary tools to achieve success; and share data. Although there are numerous models described in the literature, focusing on these 4 pillars is relatively simple and provides a good framework to building a collaborative antimicrobial stewardship initiative.

REVIEW OF PRIMARY LITERATURE ON STEWARDSHIP-HOSPITALIST INITIATIVES

Table 2 summarizes the primary literature demonstrating the impact of targeted, co-led stewardship-hospitalist interventions. Among the 12 stewardship-hospitalist

Table 1 Model for antimicrobial stewardship and hospitalist collaboration	
Primary Pillars and Indicators of Collaboration	**Description**
I. Governance • Leadership • Centrality • Support for innovation • Connectivity	• Establish coleadership among stewardship and hospitalist groups • Recommended to focus on a central goal • Provide active and ongoing communication, which should be adjusted throughout the collaboration • Provide support from both parties when implementing innovations or initiatives aimed at improving antimicrobial prescribing
II. Shared vision and goals • Goals • Patient-centered orientation and other allegiances	• Find common problem to solve and develop goals, which should always include the best interest of the patient • Discuss impact for each party involved in collaboration and identify any barriers that exist to committing to goals
III. Formalization • Information exchange • Formalization of tools	• Assign responsibilities and expectations • Develop tools to enhance communication related to expectations of each collaborator
IV. Internalization • Trust • Mutual acquaintance	• Build professional relationships through active communication • Focus on developing trust

Adapted from D'Amour D, Goulet L, Labadie JF, Martín-Rodriguez LS, Pineault R. A model and typology of collaboration between professionals in healthcare organizations. *BMC Health Serv Res.* 2008;8:1-14; with permission.

publications included in **Table 2**, about half focus on implementing initiatives aimed at broadly affecting antimicrobial prescribing.[8,9,11,16–18] These initiatives could include antimicrobial time outs; antimicrobial order forms or flowsheets; collaborative review with pharmacists or infectious disease physicians; or focused adherence to stewardship guidelines. The impact of these initiatives varies, but all report significant decreases in unnecessary antimicrobial therapy. Finally, the strategies used to implement the initiatives shared many commonalities, which include the development of written materials, education, joint review, and feedback.

The remaining studies included in **Table 2** implemented interventions that focused on specific disease states (ie, pneumonia) or focused on improving utilization of a target antimicrobial agent or antimicrobial class (ie, fluoroquinolones).[19–24] The implementation of disease-based stewardship initiatives offers the opportunity to assess the impact on clinical outcomes, in addition to antimicrobial utilization, cost, and adverse effects. Hamilton and colleagues[11] reported a decrease in mortality (0.6% vs 3.4%, $P=.008$) following implementation of a stewardship-hospitalist initiative aimed at evaluating compliance with a pneumonia-based order set. Other disease-based studies demonstrated reductions in antimicrobial therapy, without adversely affecting clinical outcomes.[19,20,22,24] With broad-based initiatives and drug-specific initiatives, it is very difficult to link changes to improvements in clinical outcomes, because the types of infections can vary significantly. Improving patient outcomes should be the ultimate goal; however, initial stewardship-hospitalist efforts should identify short-term opportunities (ie, decreasing excessive antimicrobial use) as the primary outcome.

Table 2
Review of hospitalist-led stewardship initiatives

Author	Strategy	Methods	Results
Hamilton et al,[11] 2015	• Decision support	• Multihospital pilot project. • Development of a daily flowsheet, which served as a point-of-prescription tool to assess daily antimicrobial prescribing practices. • The flowsheet was completed by a hospitalist, unit pharmacist, or nurse initiated and housestaff completed.	• 96% of patients treated with an antimicrobial agent had the flowsheet completed. • Hospitals using providers for flowsheet completion had ~5% of antimicrobial prescriptions affected. • Hospitals using pharmacists for flowsheet completion had ~40% of antimicrobial prescriptions were affected. • One hospital with pharmacist flowsheet completion reported 33 interventions on 35 patients.
Miller et al,[19] 2010	• Decision support	• Retrospective case-control study in an integrated health system. • Used evidence-based order sets for patients discharged with CAP.	• Reduction of in-hospital mortality (0.6% vs 3.4%; P value 0.008), average length of stay (4.2 d vs 4.84 d; $P = .015$), and direct cost mean ($3659 vs $4164; $P = .012$) for the order set group relative to the no order set group.
Halpape et al,[20] 2014	• Audit-feedback • Education	• Three-phased study. • Assessed a baseline and postintervention chart audit and educational intervention (audit and feedback) of local hospitalists. • Developed treatment algorithms for CAP, HAP, and HCAP, and provided education and audit results to hospitalists.	• Postintervention adherence to treatment algorithms increased from 10% to 38%. • Nonstatistically significant trend toward reduced duration of therapy in the postintervention group.
Kisuule et al,[16] 2008	• Review and feedback	• Retrospective chart review. • Assessed hospitalist-written antimicrobial prescription appropriateness (appropriate, effective but inappropriate, or inappropriate). • Hospitalists underwent a review session of inappropriate antimicrobial prescribing and practice guidelines. • Prescribing was then assessed prospectively.	• Appropriateness of antimicrobial prescriptions increased from 43% to 74% after the intervention. • Inappropriate prescriptions decreased from 57% to 26%, $P<.001$.

McGarry et al,[24] 2012	• Review and feedback • Education • Guideline development • Hospitalist-pharmacist collaboration	• Prospective cohort study at an academic medical center. • Assessed hospitalist patients with SSTIs. • Interventions included provider education through clinical conferences, SSTI guideline pocketcard development, floor pharmacist monitoring of ticarcillin/clavulanate use, and provider feedback via report cards.	• 60% decrease in time of exposure to broad-spectrum antibiotics (0.62 vs 0.25, $P = .0016$). • Decrease in the number of patients treated with 1 or more doses of excessive antibiotics (90% vs 54%, P value .0002). • Decrease in the cost of ticarcillin/clavulanate from $3189.18 to $1767.96.
Feucht et al,[21] 2003	• Education • Guideline development • Pharmacist collaboration	• Multidisciplinary, prospective interventional program at a VA Medical Center. • Utilized guidelines and monthly conferences for medical residents regarding the discontinuation of vancomycin, fluoroquinolones, and double-coverage of gram-negative bacteria with fluoroquinolones. • Clinical pharmacists prospectively reviewed new orders for appropriateness and performed interventions.	• Reduction in double gram-negative coverage by 26% ($P<.001$). • 43% decrease use of intravenous fluoroquinolones and 16% for vancomycin when administered >5 d. • Clinical pharmacist interventions had a 76% success rate.
Huang & Seymann,[22] 2009	• Education • Guideline development	• Retrospective chart review at an academic medical center. • Evaluated antibiotic selection for pneumonia within 48 h of admission. • Intervention consisted of an educational survey for HCAP guideline-recommended antimicrobials.	• Increase from 23% to 32% ($P = .03$) in the percent of patients treated with HCAP guideline-recommended antibiotics. • Decrease from 41% to 34% ($P = .13$) in the percent of patients treated for CAP. • Increase from 49% to 57% ($P = .08$) of patients prescribed at least 1 antipseudomonal agent.

(continued on next page)

Table 2
(*continued*)

Author	Strategy	Methods	Results
Mack et al,[9] 2016	• Education • Guideline development • Hospitalist-pharmacist collaboration	• Multicenter collaborative with the implementation of at least 1 of 3 strategies identified by hospitalists at a CDC kick-off meeting. • Strategies included documentation at points of care, improved clarity and accessibility of guidelines, and 72-h antimicrobial timeouts. • Clinical pharmacists collaborated with the 72-h antimicrobial timeout to determine continued antimicrobial use, treatment duration, and if the condition still required treatment.	• Complete antimicrobial documentation increased from 4% to 51% for 1 hospital and 8% to 65% for another hospital. • Optimization or discontinuation of antimicrobial agents for the 72-h timeout occurred 30% of the time.
Schwartz et al,[17] 2007	• Education • Guideline implementation	• Prospective, quasi-experimental before-and-after study in a public long-term care facility and acute care hospital. • Interventions consisted of using national guidelines, hospital resistance data, and physician feedback through teaching sessions and institutional guideline development for the treatment of common infections.	• Initial therapy with guideline recommendations was 11% in the preintervention cohort vs 39% in post (*P*<.001). • Mean census-adjusted monthly antimicrobial days decreased by 29.7%. • New starts on antimicrobials decreased by 25.9%.
Shabbir et al,[23] 2010	• Education • Guideline development	• A before-and-after study at a small metro hospital. • Intervention consisted of education on fluoroquinolone use. Used a physician champion and education was provided via newsletter and to hospital medicine physicians on the *C difficile* infection program. • Included guidelines for diverticulitis and pyelonephritis antibiotic choices. • A microbiologist performed occasional review of levofloxacin use and documentation.	• Decreased levofloxacin defined daily dose per patient hospital from 0.17 to 0.13 (*P*<.001) after education was provided.

Tang et al,[8] 2019	• Education • Hospitalist-pharmacist collaboration	• A 3-arm pre-post quality improvement study an academic medical center. • Interventions for adult internal medicine teaching services included an educational bundle, educational bundle plus antimicrobial stewardship rounds twice weekly with an infectious disease pharmacist, and educational bundle plus internal medicine-trained clinical pharmacist attending daily rounds.	• Decreased total antibiotic use by 16.8% (P<.001) in the educational bundle arm, 6.8% (P = .08) in the educational bundle plus antimicrobial stewardship rounds twice weekly with an infectious disease pharmacist arm, and 33.0% (P<.001) in the educational bundle plus internal medicine-trained clinical pharmacist attending daily rounds arm. • Decreased broad-spectrum antibiotic use of 26.2% (P<.001) in the educational bundle arm, 7.8% (P = .09) in the educational bundle plus antimicrobial stewardship rounds twice weekly with an infectious disease pharmacist arm, and 32.4% (P<.001) in the educational bundle plus internal medicine-trained clinical pharmacist attending daily rounds arm. • Decreased length of stay from 9 to 7 d in the education bundle arm and 9 to 6 d in the educational bundle plus internal medicine-trained clinical pharmacist attending daily rounds arm (P<.001 for both groups).
Yogo et al,[18] 2017	• Guideline development • Pharmacist collaboration	• Single center, quasi-experimental retrospective study. • Intervention consisted of guidance for step-down oral antibiotics and duration of therapy and discharge prescription audit by pharmacy with recommendations to providers.	• Decreased use of broad-spectrum gram-negative coverage (51% vs 40%, P = .02). • Decreased fluoroquinolone use (38% vs 25%, P = .002). • Decreased total duration of therapy from a median of 10 to 9 d (P = .13). • Decreased duration of therapy at discharge from 6 to 5 d (P = .003). • Increased overall appropriateness of therapy at discharge from 52% to 66% (P = .15).

Abbreviations: CAP, community-acquired pneumonia; CDC, Centers for Disease Control and Prevention; HAP, hospital-acquired pneumonia; HCAP, healthcare-associated pneumonia; SSTI, skin and soft tissue infection; VA, veterans affairs.

Hospitalist collaboration with other health care professionals has the potential to play a critical role in antimicrobial stewardship initiatives. Rohde and colleagues[7] identified research and quality improvement programs through the Society of Hospital Medicine abstracts to provide examples for hospitalist opportunity in antimicrobial stewardship programs (ASPs). Rosenberg discussed offering local or national high-level training programs for hospitalists on skin and soft tissue infections, pneumonia, and catheter-related infections to help promote antimicrobial stewardship, and/or partnering with infectious disease specialists to develop protocols for small ASPs within an institution.[10] Using strategies for antimicrobial stewardship at the point-of-prescription in daily practice has also been suggested.[11] This relies on decision support programs or computer assistance to provide patient-specific recommendations when an antimicrobial agent is ordered.[25] Three improvement strategies for antimicrobial use identified by hospitalists included improved documentation/visibility at points of care, improved guideline clarity and accessibility, and 72-hour antimicrobial time-outs, which have previously been described in the literature.[7,9] In addition to provider education and guideline development, other stewardship strategies include formulary restriction, which consists of the restricted dispensing of antimicrobial agents based on indication.[25]

POSITIONING HOSPITALISTS TO IMPROVE STEWARDSHIP
Laying the Foundation: What Are Key Elements to Educating Hospitalists?

How have hospitalists previously been and how will they continue to be successful stewards of antimicrobial use? Arming hospitalists with the appropriate baseline knowledge is the key first step. Educating health care providers about the importance of, and their particular role in, antimicrobial stewardship, has been an ongoing effort for almost a decade. The Centers for Disease Control and Prevention's (CDC's) "Get Smart for Healthcare" campaign in 2010 brought national attention to the connection between antimicrobial misuse and increasingly resistant pathogens, along with how curbing use could stem the tide of antimicrobial resistance and its negative downstream effects.[26] Adapting these concepts into manageable and practical educational tools are essential for frontline providers, such as hospitalists. The availability of institution-specific guidelines on commonly encountered hospital infections is a start; however, embedding these recommendations into day-to-day hospitalist workflow is a crucial next step in executing these practices. In addition, tailoring stewardship education and interventions to be based on focused, physician-specific root causes for initial underperformance is preferred to "cookie cutter" predesignated interventions based on higher-level, aggregated data. This was illustrated in a multihospital, multidepartment study using behavioral theory to affect antimicrobial appropriateness and consumption, which used behavioral principles of respect for autonomy, a sense of ownership that is self-created, and a sense of obligation to a public commitment. By identifying department-specific reasons for inappropriate prescribing, developing interventions targeted to those unique reasons, and receiving ongoing audit and feedback on performance, mean antimicrobial appropriateness was significantly increased, and the increase was sustained for greater than 12 months.[27] Thus, using a "bottom-up" rather than "top-down" approach to implementing stewardship interventions is essential to both initial and continued success.

Several studies have shown the feasibility and uptake of antimicrobial stewardship practices by frontline providers, including hospitalists, when using multimodal approaches and feedback at the point-of-care rather than retrospectively. One study used an initial education session followed by pocket cards, visual displays on patient care units, and reminders at staff meetings to reinforce documentation of antimicrobial indication and adherence to guidelines, as well as the rationale behind it. This, coupled with ongoing feedback, more than doubled providers' compliance with prescribing policy.[28] Another study targeted house staff antimicrobial prescribing by combining education around stewardship principles with online "timeout" checklists that reinforced CDC-recommended stewardship practices (ie, avoidance of broad-spectrum antimicrobials when not clinically indicated). This approach showed not only 80% adherence to "timeout" expectations, but also significant reductions in annual antimicrobial costs and rates of *Clostridium difficile* infection.[29]

Decision Support: Embedding Stewardship Practices

Understanding hospitalist workflow is key to developing successful stewardship interventions that maximize efficiency and minimize disruption. Hospitalist time-motion studies have shown that indirect patient care constitutes the most time during shifts, with electronic health record (EHR) interface being most of that time.[30] In addition, multitasking occurred during 16% of shift time, meaning that 1 task began before the completion of another, which could contribute to distractions around critical decision making.[30]

Clinical decision support systems (CDSSs) built into EHRs have the potential to enhance stewardship interventions by integrating real-time patient data into reports, alerts, and recommendations that make actionable changes more feasible. For example, current lab data, microbiology data, antibiograms, and antimicrobial use can be coupled with guideline-specific recommendations to allow for easier provider recognition and adjustment of inappropriate antimicrobial use. Several CDSSs have been designed specifically for ASPs.[31] Stewardship-focused CDSSs have been shown to increase acceptance of stewardship interventions, specifically decreasing use of overly broad antimicrobials, antimicrobials in noninfectious conditions, and duplicate antimicrobial coverage; however, this does come with the consequence of added time spent receiving and reviewing alerts[32] This so-called alert fatigue can result in providers overriding or dismissing important clinical decision making opportunities when inundated with alerts of varying priority and relevance. In addition, there are significant financial costs with initiation and maintenance of CDSSs, as well as provider perception of loss of control and autonomy in antimicrobial prescribing. All of these factors have driven further work into developing more user-friendly, less costly CDSSs by engaging the end-user (hospitalist and/or resident physicians) in their development. One study engaged frontline providers, including hospitalists, in the CDSS design of data visualization for early recognition of antimicrobial-resistant organisms, as well as appropriate antimicrobial selection in easily viewable formats. They also recommended alerts be persuasive rather than restrictive.[33] Real-time availability of integrated clinical information, appropriate alerts, and the downstream multidisciplinary communication were all recognized as advantages to the CDSS and a reflection of direct end-user involvement from concept to execution. Another study used a low-fidelity CDSS prototype and hypothetical clinical scenarios to query resident physicians about what clinical data should be viewable and other diagnostic testing to be pursued, with secondary input from experts of various specialties.[34] The authors described discordance in opinion among experts within the same specialty when choosing relevant displayed data and recommendations for further testing. This highlights that, although all stakeholders may not agree on the details, a CDSS should support frontline providers in the clinical decision making process rather than dictating a one-size-fits-all directive.[34] Having hospitalists act in this advisory role has the potential to create useful, efficient, and noninterruptive antimicrobial stewardship CDSSs.

Hospitalists as Stewardship Champions

Hospitalists cannot only be successful practitioners of stewardship tenets and developers of effective decision support but can also lead the charge as antimicrobial stewardship champions. CDC issued a call to arms for hospitalist-led stewardship in 2011[35] by recognizing their unique position as primary prescribers for a significant amount of antimicrobials, their quality improvement experience, and the sheer number and presence of hospitalists at institutions of all sizes across the country. Successful stewardship initiatives need not require expertise from stewardship-specialized infectious disease physicians or pharmacists because these roles may not exist in smaller community hospitals. Hamilton and colleagues[11] evaluated the feasibility of a point-of-care antimicrobial prescribing rounding tool that was implemented in 4 different hospitals, all of which did not have existing stewardship programs. A variety of providers, including hospitalists, tested the rounding tool and found it to be easy and quick, with variability in prompting change of antimicrobial. The authors stressed that point-of-care interventions have the ability to identify stewardship opportunities not otherwise apparent by an external team not directly involved in the patient's care. Hospitalists can provide a unique connection between broadly applicable stewardship principles and the nuances of day-to-day patient-specific scenarios and have done so without formal stewardship oversight.

Mack and colleagues[9] describe the successful hospitalist-led implementation of 3 key strategies (standard antimicrobial use documentation, accessible guidelines, and instituting an antimicrobial timeout) in 5 diverse hospitals. By adapting interventions into each hospital medicine program's unique workflow, frequent check-ins to discuss successes and challenges at each hospital, and hospitalist leaders "modeling" stewardship practices themselves, almost a 10-fold improvement was seen in 2 hospitals with complete antimicrobial use documentation (indication, day of therapy, and duration). In addition, the institution completing antimicrobial timeouts resulted in de-escalation or discontinuation of antimicrobials 30% of the time, which may not have otherwise occurred.[9] When stewardship-hospitalist champions are coupled with clinical pharmacists on multidisciplinary rounds that occur regularly, stewardship practices are not only embedded in daily practice but showcased for trainees and other medical providers. The regular occurrence of rounds and stewardship discussions may be as, if not more, important than dedicated infectious disease-trained pharmacists. Tang and colleagues[8] found that hospitalist team rounding with internal medicine-trained pharmacists that occurred on an almost daily basis had a greater impact on total antimicrobial and broad-spectrum antimicrobial usage than twice weekly rounding with infectious disease-trained pharmacists. Thus, the frequent role modeling of hospitalist and pharmacy stewardship discussions may be more impactful on important stewardship outcomes than specialty training of either the physician or the pharmacist, which can be adapted to settings in which formal stewardship trained specialists may not exist.[8] Implementing a hospitalist-driven stewardship initiative, however, is not without challenges.

Table 3 summarizes barriers and potential countermeasures to hospitalist-led stewardship initiatives.

Using Clinical Pharmacists

The role of a pharmacist can differ based on organizational needs and structure: the individual pharmacist involved in the ASP may range from a frontline pharmacist

Table 3
Barriers and countermeasures to implementing stewardship initiatives

Barrier	Potential Countermeasure
Overly general "top-down" stewardship approaches	Modifying interventions and targeting goals to address hospitalist-specific deficiencies Advocating for hospitalist participation on institutional stewardship committees
Stewardship awareness and education	Multimodal, ongoing education sessions using hospitalist-focused examples (ie, group conferences, visual reminders)
Lack of peer engagement	Identifying a hospitalist stewardship champion that sets the example for group ("walking the walk") Providing individualized, real-time feedback to underperformers
Dissemination and uptake of stewardship tools	Partnering of hospitalist with informatics to develop nonintrusive clinical decision support systems in the electronic medical record Embedding stewardship checklist usage in multidisciplinary rounds
Validating importance of initial stewardship successes	Incentivizing stewardship-driven outcomes with group and/or individual bonuses Publicizing hospitalist successes at the institution level

performing order verification to an informatics-trained pharmacist developing automated alerts for providers or other pharmacists.[36,37] There are many different initiatives for infectious disease-trained pharmacists to get involved with; however, like many aspects in health care, resources and availability of infectious disease-trained pharmacists may be limited. A potential solution for this is to engage and train other members of the pharmacy team who are not formally infectious disease trained. This may include pharmacy learners, such as pharmacy residents or pharmacy students, as it is important to recognize these individuals as essential members of the ASP team.[38] Furthermore, infectious disease-trained pharmacists can provide these pharmacy team members with the framework and support to be successful. An additional way to expand the reach of ASP programs is to involve multiple medical centers where institutions without ASP programs and/or trained pharmacists could seek out collaboration with institutions that have ASP pharmacists.[39–41]

With the advancement of the EHR, the possibilities and opportunities for automated alerts and reports are endless. Noninfectious disease-trained pharmacists can be quickly alerted to real-time bacteremia results, patients with inappropriately labeled antimicrobial allergies, bug-drug mismatches, procalcitonin results, or more straightforward interventions, such as intravenous to oral conversions or renal function dosing adjustments. Working with a well-equipped informatics-trained pharmacist and developing these tools allows for pharmacists to be more efficient, engaging in a wider scope of practice and handling a larger patient load.

Development of policies that allow pharmacists to be able to automatically implement changes to patients' medication therapy increases efficiency and offloads hospitalists' work; however, there will remain clinical scenarios that dictate direct peer-to-peer discussion with the primary team. A strong pharmacist-hospitalist relationship can allow ASP programs to truly excel. Having an open line of communication is vital, as is having devoted time in a busy day to spend discussing medication therapy plans. It has been documented that these protected antimicrobial discussions, or time outs, can lead to a decrease in antimicrobial use and an increase in antimicrobial optimization.[9] These daily discussions can also allow for the pharmacist to discuss stewardship updates including but not limited to new formulary restrictions, guideline revisions, antibiogram updates, or historical *C difficile* infection rates.

SUMMARY

Optimizing antimicrobial prescribing requires efforts outside the ASP and should be a responsibility of all health care providers. Hospitalists are ideal collaborators, as they treat a large percentage of hospitalized patients admitted with infection. In addition, they are increasingly engaged in quality improvement activities and clinical research, skills that dovetail into affecting and leading stewardship efforts. Finally, hospitalists play an important role in mentoring medical, pharmacy, and nursing trainees, and can shape the perceptions of antimicrobial stewardship to a diverse group of learners. The importance of developing good stewardship-hospitalist collaboration cannot be overstated.

DISCLOSURE

The authors did not receive funding for this work or have any conflicts of interest to disclose.

REFERENCES

1. Wachter RM, Goldman L. Zero to 50,000—the 20th anniversary of the hospitalist. N Engl J Med 2016;375(11):1009–11.
2. Landrigan CP, Conway PH, Edwards S, et al. Pediatric hospitalists: a systematic review of the literature. Pediatrics 2006;117(5):1736–44.
3. McCarthy MW, Walsh TJ. The rise of hospitalists: an opportunity for infectious diseases investigators. Expert Rev Anti Infect Ther 2018;16(5):385–9.
4. Townsend J, Gundareddy VP, Zenilman JM. Project step in: stewardship through education of providers in the inpatient setting lead editor: Editors: implementation guide to establish antimicrobial stewardship practices among hospitalists and other hospitalist clinicians. Available at: www.hospitalmedicine.org/ABX. Accessed December 26, 2019.
5. Fridkin S, Baggs J, Fagan R, et al. Vital signs: improving antibiotic use among hospitalized patients. Morb Mortal Wkly Rep 2014;63:9.
6. Kelesidis T, Braykov N, Uslan DZ, et al. Indications and types of antibiotic agents used in 6 acute care: a pragmatic retrospective observational study. Infect Control Hosp Epidemiol 2016;37(1):70–9.
7. Rohde JM, Jacobsen D, Rosenberg DJ. Role of the hospitalist in antimicrobial stewardship: a review of work completed and description of a multisite collaborative. Clin Ther 2013;35(6):751–7.
8. Tang SJ, Gupta R, Lee JI, et al. Impact of hospitalist-led interdisciplinary antimicrobial stewardship interventions at an academic medical center. Jt Comm J Qual Patient Saf 2019;45(3):207–16.
9. Mack MR, Rohde JM, Jacobsen D, et al. Engaging hospitalists in antimicrobial stewardship: lessons from a multihospital collaborative. J Hosp Med 2016; 11(8):576–80.
10. Rosenberg DJ. Infections, bacterial resistance, and antimicrobial stewardship: the emerging role of hospitalists. J Hosp Med 2012;7(SUPPL. 1):S34–43.

11. Hamilton KW, Gerber JS, Moehring R, et al. Point-of-prescription interventions to improve antimicrobial stewardship. Clin Infect Dis 2015;60(8):1252–8.
12. Dellit TH. Summary of the Infectious Diseases Society of America and the Society for Healthcare Epidemiology of America guidelines for developing an institutional program to enhance antimicrobial stewardship. Infect Dis Clin Pract (Baltim Md) 2007;15(4):263–4.
13. New_Antimicrobial_Stewardship_Standard.
14. Karam M, Brault I, Van Durme T, et al. Comparing interprofessional and interorganizational collaboration in healthcare: a systematic review of the qualitative research. Int J Nurs Stud 2018;79(November 2017):70–83.
15. D'Amour D, Goulet L, Labadie JF, et al. A model and typology of collaboration between professionals in healthcare organizations. BMC Health Serv Res 2008; 8:1–14.
16. Kisuule F, Wright S, Barreto J, et al. Improving antibiotic utilization among hospitalists: a pilot academic detailing project with a public health approach. J Hosp Med 2008;3(1):64–70. Abstract Available at: https://www.ncbi.nlm.nih.gov/pubmed/18257048.
17. Schwartz DN, Abiad H, DeMarais PL, et al. An educational intervention to improve antimicrobial use in a hospital-based long-term care facility. J Am Geriatr Soc 2007;55(8):1236–42.
18. Yogo N, Shihadeh K, Young H, et al. Intervention to reduce broad-spectrum antibiotics and treatment durations prescribed at the time of hospital discharge: a novel stewardship approach. Infect Control Hosp Epidemiol 2017;38(5):534–41.
19. Miller S, Bognani S, Phillips K, et al. Implementation of evidence-based order sets improves clinical and financial outcomes in the treatment of pneumonia and heart failure [Abstract]. J Hosp Med 2010;5(suppl 1). Abstract Available at: https://www.shmabstracts.com/abstract/implementation-of-ev.
20. Halpape K, Sulz L, Schuster B, et al. Audit and feedback-focused approach to evidence-based care in treating patients with pneumonia in hospital (AFFECT Study). Can J Hosp Pharm 2014;67(1):17–27.
21. Feucht CL, Rice LB. An interventional program to improve antibiotic use [Abstract]. Ann Pharmacother 2003;37(5):646–51. Abstract Available at: https://journals.sagepub.com/doi/10.1345/aph.1C166.
22. Huang B, Seymann G. Increased utilization of guideline-recommended antibiotics for health care-associated pneumonia following an educational intervention [Abstract]. J Hosp Med 2009;4(suppl 1):47. Abstract Available at: https://www.shmabstracts.com/abstract/increased-utilizati.
23. Shabbir H, Stone J, Singh A, et al. Hospital medicine education program reduces fluoroquinolone use [Abstract]. J Hosp Med 2010;5(suppl 1):130. Abstract Available at: https://www.shmabstracts.com/abstract/hospital-medicine-education-program-reduces-floroquinolone-use/.
24. McGarry M, Alvarez K, Kannan S, et al. Antimicrobial stewardship on the hospitalist service: skin and soft tissue infections [Abstract]. J Hosp Med 2012; 7(suppl 2):55. Abstract Available at: https://www.shmabstracts.com/abstract/antimicrobial-stewardship-on-the-hospitalist-service-skin-and-so.
25. MacDougall C, Polk RE. Antimicrobial stewardship programs in health care systems. Clin Microbiol Rev 2005;18(4):638–56.
26. Get Smart for Healthcare. Implementation resources. Available at: www.cdc.gov/getsmart/healthcare/implementation.html.
27. Sikkens JJ, Van Agtmael MA, Peters EJG, et al. Behavioral approach to appropriate antimicrobial prescribing in hospitals the Dutch unique method for

antimicrobial stewardship (DUMAS) participatory intervention study. JAMA Intern Med 2017;177(8):1130–8.

28. Thakkar K, Gilchrist M, Dickinson E, et al. A quality improvement programme to increase compliance with an anti-infective prescribing policy. J Antimicrob Chemother 2011;66(8):1916–20.

29. Lee TC, Frenette C, Jayaraman D, et al. Antibiotic self-stewardship: trainee-led structured antibiotic time-outs to improve antimicrobial use. Ann Intern Med 2014;161:S53–8.

30. Tipping MD, Forth VE, O'Leary KJ, et al. Where did the day go? A time-motion study of hospitalists. J Hosp Med 2010;5(6):323–8.

31. Kullar R, Goff DA. Transformation of antimicrobial stewardship programs through technology and informatics. Infect Dis Clin North Am 2014;28(2):291–300.

32. Hermsen ED, Vanschooneveld TC, Sayles H, et al. Implementation of a clinical decision support system for antimicrobial stewardship. Infect Control Hosp Epidemiol 2012;33(4):412–5. Special Topic Issue: Published by: Cambridge University Press.

33. Simões AS, Maia MR, Gregório J, et al. Participatory implementation of an antibiotic stewardship programme supported by an innovative surveillance and clinical decision-support system. J Hosp Infect 2018;100:257–64.

34. Beerlage-de Jong N, Wentzel J, Hendrix R, et al. The value of participatory development to support antimicrobial stewardship with a clinical decision support system. Am J Infect Control 2017;45(4):365–71.

35. Srinivasan A. Engaging hospitalists in antimicrobial stewardship: the CDC perspective. J Hosp Med 2011;6(Suppl 1):S31–3.

36. Laible BR, Nazir J, Assimacopoulos AP, et al. Implementation of a pharmacist-led antimicrobial management team in a community teaching hospital: use of pharmacy residents and pharmacy students in a prospective audit and feedback approach. J Pharm Pract 2010;23(6):531–5.

37. Carreno JJ, Kenney RM, Bloome M, et al. Evaluation of pharmacy generalists performing antimicrobial stewardship services. Am J Health Syst Pharm 2015; 72(15):1298–303.

38. Chahine EB, El-Lababidi RM, Sourial M. Engaging pharmacy students, residents, and fellows in antimicrobial stewardship. J Pharm Pract 2015;28(6):585–91.

39. Waters CD. Pharmacist-driven antimicrobial stewardship program in an institution without infectious diseases physician support. Am J Health Syst Pharm 2015; 72(6):466–8.

40. Dubrovskaya Y, Scipione MR, Siegfried J, et al. Multilayer model of pharmacy participation in the antimicrobial stewardship program at a large academic medical center. Hosp Pharm 2017;52(9):628–34.

41. Crader M. Development of antimicrobial competencies and training for staff hospital pharmacists. Hosp Pharm 2014;49(1):32–41.

Collaborative Antimicrobial Stewardship for Surgeons

Evan D. Robinson, MD[a], David F. Volles, Pharm D, BCCCP[b], Katherine Kramme, DO[c], Amy J. Mathers, MD, D(ABMM)[a], Robert G. Sawyer, MD[c],*

KEYWORDS

- Surgery • Antibiotic stewardship • Antimicrobial resistance

KEY POINTS

- Optimal antimicrobial stewardship involving surgeons works best when collaboration is open.
- Each involved party (surgeons, infectious diseases experts, and pharmacists) have important specialized knowledge to contribute.
- Evidence-based practices are at the core of cooperation between all members of the antimicrobial stewardship effort.

Although antibiotics represent one of the most important therapeutic modalities used by the modern health care provider, antibiotic misuse, abuse, and the consequences thereof, including the rise of multidrug-resistant organisms, represents one of the most pressing public health concerns worldwide. Antibiotic exposure is the risk factor most strongly linked with the development of resistant infections,[1–4] with some studies estimating the rate of inappropriate antibiotic prescribing patterns to be as high as 50%.[5,6] The current trajectory of antimicrobial resistance is reversible, however, this reversal can only take place with concentrated efforts to minimize inappropriate antibiotic exposure.[7] Formal antimicrobial stewardship programs are increasing in popularity in an effort to address this crisis.

The Infectious Disease Society of America and Society for Healthcare Epidemiology of America guidelines identify 2 core evidence-based strategies for promoting stewardship. These include the utilization of preprescription authorization (PPA) for certain antimicrobials and/or postprescription review with feedback (PPRF) to antimicrobial prescribers, in addition to supplemental strategies, such as provider education, and intravenous to parenteral transition protocols.[8] Although there is conflicting data regarding superiority of one approach over the other, data consistently suggest that

[a] Department of Medicine, Division of Infectious Diseases, University of Virginia, PO Box 801340, Charlottesville, VA 22908-1340, USA; [b] Department of Pharmacy, University of Virginia, PO Box 800674, Charlottesville, VA 22908, USA; [c] Department of Surgery, Western Michigan University Homer Stryker MD School of Medicine, 1000 Oakland Drive, Kalamazoo, MI 49008, USA
* Corresponding author.
E-mail address: robert.sawyer@med.wmich.edu

Infect Dis Clin N Am 34 (2020) 97–108
https://doi.org/10.1016/j.idc.2019.11.002
0891-5520/20/© 2019 Elsevier Inc. All rights reserved.

id.theclinics.com

formal implementation of antimicrobial stewardship programs improves appropriate antibiotic selection and decreases duration of antibiotic therapy.[7,9–12] Although these studies rarely report a difference in clinical outcome, a significant cost reduction is seen.[9,13–15]

Of particular interest is not just the establishment of antibiotic stewardship programs, but the engagement of the prescribing clinicians, particularly surgeons. Surgeons have a unique role to play as the frequent prescriber of both prophylactic and therapeutic antimicrobials. However, literature to date suggests surgeon compliance with evidence-based antibiotic guidelines is low.[5,16,17] This begs the question— What is the most effective way to ensure faithful antibiotic stewardship practices among surgeons? Obviously, opinions about best practices may depend on the point of view of the specialty of the clinician involved in the antimicrobial stewardship team-surgeon collaboration. The following is a multidisciplinary discussion including a clinical pharmacist, infectious disease specialists, and surgeons in an attempt to answer that very question.

ROLE OF THE PHARMACIST IN ANTIMICROBIAL STEWARDSHIP WORKING WITH SURGEONS

Antibiotic stewardship is especially important on surgical wards where up to half the prescriptions for antibiotics have been assessed to be inappropriate based on some component of therapy including selection of agent based on indication, dose, or duration. In addition, surgical patients are particularly vulnerable to infectious complications as they have been found to have a higher mortality than for similar complications in nonsurgical patients.[18] It does appear that the Surgical Quality Improvement Project has improved the use of antimicrobials for surgical prophylaxis with perhaps a small decrease in rates of surgical site infection,[19] yet with the ongoing improper antibiotic use involving use of antibiotics without a solid indication, use of an agent with inappropriate antimicrobial coverage, or failure to discontinue antibiotics on resolution of the infection.

All members of the health care team have the important goal of improving utilization of antimicrobial agents within the health system, however, pharmacists have a unique role working with all other members of the team including surgeons and infectious diseases physicians, gaining consensus and oftentimes bridging gaps of opinions between different members of the team regarding the best course of action. Pharmacist's roles and justification for pharmacist roles with antibiotic stewardship initially had been focused on cost containment activities, however, they have evolved into working directly with patient care teams, providing high-level care and recommendations that improve quality and safety. Pharmacists develop strong working relationships with members of the surgery teams and are in a good position to make recommendations regarding changes in therapy which are often accepted by surgery team members leading to improved patient outcomes. Generally speaking, stewardship interventions are more effective when one can take a nonthreatening approach to collaboration, and in our experience, pharmacists frequently fill this role. In addition, pharmacists view their role as providing a safety net ensuring safe, appropriate use of antibiotics. Pharmacists are very dependent on interdisciplinary collaboration that enables good communication with other teams and also may encourage involvement from the infectious diseases experts when appropriate. Pharmacists with their involvement in clinical practice on surgical wards, both acute care and critical care, are in a good position to provide a daily medication profile review looking for opportunities for improvements in the use of antibiotics. Pharmacists are not necessarily the deciders for many of these complex issues, such as the presence or absence of infection or appropriate timing of de-escalation, however, they are the health care providers who are in a position to bring up questions and recommendations regarding antibiotic use in a safe noncritical environment. Pharmacist's interventions with antimicrobial use generally focus on appropriate drug selection based on antibiotic coverage and need for broad versus a narrow spectrum, appropriate dose using pharmacokinetic and pharmacodynamics principles, appropriate route considering intravenous versus oral, and duration of therapy.

OPPORTUNITIES IN EMPIRIC THERAPY

In general, broad-spectrum agents should be initiated for the decompensating patient or certain specific situations, such as complicated skin structure infections, and properly include coverage for resistant gram-positive organisms, such as methicillin-resistant *Staphylococcus aureus* (MRSA). Unfortunately, vancomycin and other MRSA therapies are frequently not discontinued once it becomes clear the patient does not or is not likely to have MRSA. The use of MRSA screening for colonization should be used to encourage discontinuation of MRSA therapies when it is an unlikely organism. In addition, the use of MRSA screening for patients with suspected pneumonia where it has become more common, it can also be used for patients with other suspected infections, such as severe intra-abdominal infections. A negative MRSA swab has been demonstrated to have a good negative predictive value even for intra-abdominal infections which may be due to a low incidence of MRSA in this patient population.[20] Use of unnecessary "double gram negative" coverage, double anaerobe coverage or use of antifungals without an indication are other potential sources of unnecessary antibiotic use in surgical patients and should be evaluated. In addition to appropriate spectrum, duration of antibiotic treatment should be addressed every day although the use of an antibiotic "time out" where the infection being treated is identified along with an appropriate duration for that infection. This daily antibiotic time out is a good opportunity to also address any possibility for antibiotic de-escalation if it is clear the isolated organisms are susceptible to less broad-spectrum agents.

In summary, as the medication experts, pharmacists can play an essential role improving use of antimicrobial therapy providing a safety net and improving quality of care. Leveraging good working relationships with surgery teams, pharmacists are in a good position to positively influence patient outcomes through optimization of antibiotic selection, dosing using pharmacokinetic/pharmacodynamic principles, and duration by encouraging an antibiotic time out each day. Antibiotic optimization will only continue to get more complicated with increasing resistance and with new broad-spectrum agents released to the market necessitating the ongoing role of pharmacists in antimicrobial stewardship activities.

INSIDE THE MIND OF AN INFECTIOUS DISEASE PHYSICIAN ANTIMICROBIAL STEWARDSHIP DIRECTOR

Infectious disease (ID) physicians pride themselves on being excellent internists taking the whole patient in mind. In fact, thinking about the whole patient as well as working across specialties are both frequently stated reasons for choosing the field. With that being said, when ID physicians make recommendations about antibiotic escalation/de-escalation, they are not just considering antimicrobial resources and resistance, but also the risk of toxicity including acute kidney injury and *Clostridioides difficile* infection, as well as the risk of inadequately treated infection.

From the perspective of an ID physician, working with surgeons can be challenging and rewarding. Bidirectional open, honest and data-driven dialogue is central to effective collaboration between ID and surgery. It is important to note that there are often misconceptions about the goals and aims of a stewardship program from surgeons. Misunderstanding may have arisen from a natural tension around autonomy and the important need for a surgeon to be decisive. However, stewardship and surgery have the shared goals of improving outcomes for the individual surgical patient as the highest priority. Antimicrobial stewardship is defined as "selecting the most appropriate drug at its optimal dose and duration of therapy to eradicate an infection while minimizing toxicity and impact on selective pressure."[21] However, antimicrobials are not without toxicity and side effects in the individual patient, such as C difficile infection, renal failure or allergic reactions. For many years antimicrobials were viewed as harmless and when there is diagnostic uncertainty in a clinical situation there can often be the perception of little downside to giving more antimicrobials until it is clear that the infection or even the perceived risk of infection has passed. We now know that "more is (not always) better" when it comes to antimicrobials. The goal of optimized antimicrobial stewardship programs is patient centered and not measured in cost reductions. Depending on how the stewardship program is implemented individual patient as the highest priority can be lost in messaging and sometimes in reality. However, a good stewardship program should be known for both adding appropriate antimicrobials when needed as well as suggesting removal of unnecessary antimicrobials. Between 15% and 30% of interventions in stewardship are related to adding effective antimicrobials to a regimen when a patient is on inadequate therapy rather that the concept that antimicrobial stewardship interventions merely remove, consolidate or deescalate therapy.[22,23]

INFECTIOUS DISEASES ADVICE TO SURGICAL COLLEAGUES

Preserving antimicrobials is critical to the general practice of safe surgery. For example, from a preantibiotic era series (1933–1947) of 561 patients who underwent transuretheral resection of the prostate, 6 died of sepsis and 1 from agranulocytosis from sulfadiazine.[24] To safely practice surgery, transplant and generally modern medicine we need to use and maintain effective antimicrobials. To accomplish this goal it will take a multidisciplinary approach where everyone is listening and understanding each other's perspective. As pointed out by the surgeons below, open and honest communication is required by both stewardship and surgical physicians. However, with increases in antimicrobial resistance, many agents are losing their efficacy in the setting of modern day bacteria and it is critical that we learn to effectively work together to preserve agents for future successful surgeries. Even at large hospital systems with antibiotic stewardship programs, significant amounts of surgical patients were found to be treated with too broad a regimen, and beyond the recommended duration.[5]

Antibiotic stewardship programs have been found to reduce antibiotic use, improve patient outcomes, reduce rates of C difficile infection and antibiotic resistance and lower costs.[25,26] Studies have shown conflicting results and not clearly demonstrated which of PPA or PPRF is the most effective method of implementing antibiotic stewardship.[10,12] A combination of both is likely best depending on each hospital/units resources and restriction still does play an important role for certain agents.

THERAPEUTIC

With many of the advances in modern medicine patients have become older, more immunosuppressed and generally more complicated than when antimicrobials originally came to practice. There has also been increases in antimicrobial resistance. This makes the use of antimicrobials more challenging and nuanced and potentially using the same 2 or 3 agents for all infections may no longer be been increases in antimicrobial resistance. This makes the use of antimicrobials more challenging and nuanced and potentially using the same 2 or 3 agents for all infections may no longer be effective. Although the general opinion of antimicrobial stewardship is to limit unnecessary antimicrobials it is important to note that a primary task is to recommend active antimicrobial agents when ineffective antimicrobials are in use. There are also several new antibacterial agents coming to market to combat antibiotic resistance and their use can be challenging with some advanced knowledge around specific resistance mechanisms. IDs will need to work with surgeons to help manage vulnerable patients to make sure more complicated antimicrobials are accessed when need.

PROPHYLAXIS

Use of antibiotics for surgical prophylaxis have been estimated to make up 15% of all antibiotic agents used in hospitals in point prevalence surveys.[27] Antibiotic prophylaxis has been shown in numerous studies to play a clear role along with other perioperative infection prevention measures in reducing surgical site infections (SSIs).[28] For most procedures, continued antibiotics outside the operating room have not been shown to provide benefit, and are probably associated with adverse outcomes.[29,30] However, multiple studies of adherence to published guidelines suggest compliance rates to be below 50%, with prolonged duration and inappropriate regimens commonly observed.[31,32] In addition, with the rise of antibiotic resistance there is concern for diminished effectiveness of antibiotic prophylaxis, with 1 recent meta-analysis showing a significant increase in SSIs after colorectal surgery treated with currently recommended prophylaxis regimens.[33] Stewardship could help to adjust institutional antimicrobial prophylaxis in the setting of increasing or changing resistance patterns for more effective prophylaxis.

FROM THE MIND OF A SURGEON: WHERE SURGEONS AND ANTIMICROBIAL STEWARDSHIP INTERACT

It is obvious that surgeons have a specific subset of antimicrobial uses compared with physicians in general, and that this fact influences their relationship with antimicrobial stewardship. The 3 major decision points for surgeons using antimicrobials are related to surgical prophylaxis, initiation of antimicrobials (choice and dose) for patients with known or suspected surgical infections, and definitive management of antimicrobials once an infection is diagnosed and culture results return. How and when decisions about these 3 situations are made differ significantly. Prophylaxis is typically discussed in a quiet conference room with an abundance of literature and guidelines leading to agreement. The initiation of empiric therapy, however, occurs at a more rapid pace, frequently in off-hours, especially with sepsis and septic shock guidelines demanding treatment within 1 hour. Antimicrobial management, including de-escalation and duration, can be discussed in in a few brief moments, integrated in to the daily flow of clinical care.

One special circumstance where surgeons use and misuse antimicrobials frequently, in our experience, is in the management of critically ill patients in the intensive care unit (ICU). Although many physicians equate critical illness with the Medical ICU, in hospitals with active trauma, transplant, cardiothoracic surgery, and neurosurgical programs, most patients in ICUs may be on surgical services. In addition, surgical ICUs manage a large number of nonsurgical infections, including the entire panoply of nosocomial conditions: ventilator-associated pneumonia, urinary tract infections, catheter-associated bloodstream infections, and other device-related infections. Those infections, unfortunately, occur in patients who often have other reasons to have systemic inflammation (eg, trauma, burns) with a high risk of death and increased susceptibility to drug toxicity, have conflicting diagnostic criteria (ventilator-associated pneumonia), and are caused by pathogens with high rates of antimicrobial resistance, making antimicrobial management especially challenging. In our experience, the most contentious interactions with antimicrobial stewardship teams have been related to the management of critically ill patients with significant signs of infection yet unclear diagnostic testing. We have previously demonstrated that most diagnostic criteria for sepsis lose their specificity among surgical patients treated in the ICU.[34] Because of this, decisions for initiating antimicrobials are often made with modest and inaccurate clinical criteria, such as changes in quality and quantity of sputum in a mechanically ventilated patient and 1 eye on the sepsis bundle care clock.

DEEP INSIDE THE MIND OF A SURGEON

At present, surgeons are less likely than nonsurgeons to comply with stewardship recommendations.[16] To maximize teamwork between surgeons and members of the antimicrobial stewardship team, it is probably useful to state the attitude most surgeons have about their patients and how it may influence desired antimicrobial therapy. First, once you have had your hands (or instruments) inside the body of another human, a unique personal relationship exists. Even a relatively simple operation consists of hundreds of decisions (eg, bovie or tie?), all that can change the results of a procedure and for which the surgeon feels responsible. Second, outcomes from surgery are highly scrutinized by departments, hospitals, oversight agencies, and state and federal governments. In many states it is easier to find the surgical site infection rate for an individual surgeon than it is to determine the mortality for a hospital's patients admitted with community-acquired pneumonia. Third, consistency is a key driver of efficient surgery. Experienced surgeons who are performing an operation with the same methods, instruments, and staff that they have used hundreds of times before do the most technically flawless operations (seek them out for you and your family). As a result, surgeons feel intensely responsible for their patients and are unlikely to deviate from their usual successful practices, even over an entire career. If a surgeon was taught as a resident to irrigate the abdomen with bacitracin in the setting of diffuse peritonitis, for example, as long as they believe their outcomes are superior, it is nearly impossible to convince them otherwise. Moreover, surgeons have rarely been accused of lacking self-confidence.

A result of these attitudes is an intense focus on the individual patient rather than groups of patients or environmental epidemiology; the implications for stewardship practices are obvious. Surgeons tend to be more likely to start antibiotics (which are felt to be relatively risk-free), use broader spectrum agents, and continue agents for prolonged periods, with less concern for inducing antimicrobial resistance. Consequently, surgeons tend to see proponents of stewardship to be overly concerned with antimicrobial resistance, at the expense of the individual patient. Strategically, therefore, the best way to work with surgeons is to emphasize the benefits of any intervention on the individual patient. Pointing out that an overlong course of antimicrobials puts their individual patient at risk for developing a resistant superinfection, for example, will be more convincing than any argument about changes in unit or environmental flora.

SURGEONS' THOUGHTS ABOUT INFECTIOUS DISEASES SPECIALISTS

The practices of surgery and IDs contrast in several ways, as do their practitioners. For most health care episodes that include an operation, the surgeon serves as the primary caregiver, overseeing all aspects of the care of the patient with appropriate input from others (although this model is changing over time). The surgeon integrates expertise from themselves and others, the patient's current condition, course, and trajectory, and an incredible amount of objective (although sometimes inconsistent) data to decide on the best care for the patient. On the other hand, IDs specialists are usually in a consultative role and because of that may be new to the case and only see the patient daily, may be perceived incorrectly as focusing solely on the IDs aspects of care, although they frequently have the best understanding of complex, nonsurgical medical comorbidities. Surgeons, therefore, rightly or wrongly may believe their opinion should count more than those of the "itinerant" consultant. Members of standalone antimicrobial stewardship teams that actively monitor antimicrobial prescription are in an even more difficult position, frequently accused of just reading the electronic record and making recommendations based solely on culture results and frequently inaccurate electronic documentation. In either case, working with surgeons is easiest when it is clear that the IDs specialist is considering the whole patient. It is far easier, for example, for a stewardship member to convince a surgeon to stop antimicrobials after the treatment of an intra-abdominal infection if they know and point out that normal bowel function has resumed.

One aspect of surgical infections that frequently differentiates them from medical infections is the need for a mechanical intervention for successful treatment. The major difference, for example, between treating pneumonia and a mature empyema (both thoracic infections) is the need for surgical drainage and decortication for empyema. Indeed, for many infections the most important antimicrobial-related question that must be asked of a surgeon is "Do you think you have adequate source control?" (look them in the eye when you ask). Now, contemplate the following question: Who is the expert in treating empyema, the surgeon or the infectious disease specialist? Because there is only modest overlap between skillsets, the answer is probably neither or both; both parties need to appreciate and acknowledge the expertise of each. An excellent communication with a surgeon would be "Now that you have gotten source control and it's MSSA, we can de-escalate to nafcillin." A poor communication would be "Stop the vanco."

SURGEONS' THOUGHTS ABOUT PHARMACISTS

Simply put, surgeons love pharmacists. Surgeons view pharmacists as the authorities on subjects that surgeons freely acknowledge are outside of their standard skillsets (eg, new agents, pharmacokinetics, toxicities, interactions). Childish as it may seem, interactions with pharmacists are mainly low-key, since surgeons rarely consider pharmacists confrontational or intimidating. Hence, recommendations from pharmacists are probably more likely to be accepted by surgeons, since pharmacists are seen as experts on *drugs* (where surgeons are not). In addition, the inclusion of regular pharmacist input even on ward surgery patients has long been known to significantly improve antimicrobial use.[35] Our experience suggests that a well-trained pharmacist on an antimicrobial stewardship team is an invaluable asset, and that their interactions with surgeons are frequently the key to optimizing antimicrobial use.

SUMMARY

Surgeons have many important points of contact with antimicrobial stewardship. In general, they are intensely concerned about the outcomes of their specific patients and will do almost anything they believe will improve their prognosis with less concern about population-based issues, such as antimicrobial resistance. A fruitful, collaborative relationship can be built between surgeons and the multidisciplinary antimicrobial stewardship team based on education, mutual respect, and a willingness to compromise. Practical advice from years of interactions can be found below.

ADVICE TO SURGEONS FROM INFECTIOUS DISEASE SPECIALISTS

- Optimize antimicrobial usage by shortening courses for diagnoses where data are available (eg, intra-abdominal infection), stopping empiric antimicrobials when cultures negative, and readdressing antimicrobial therapy every day with a plan for discontinuation
- Engage with the stewardship team for guidance in interpreting clinical microbiology results
- Recognize the natural history of postoperative patients as infection and recovery from surgery can often appear clinically similar, that is, sterile versus infectious inflammation, and treat infections not anxiety (eg, aspiration)
- Drain infected fluid when indicated and/or possible
- Participating in the creation of local surgical site infection prophylaxis protocols and follow them

Target therapy when possible by narrowing when cultures/susceptibility available, knowing the guidelines/local susceptibility for empiric antimicrobials for common conditions, and knowing who is at risk for multidrug-resistant infections.

ADVICE TO INFECTIOUS DISEASE SPECIALISTS FROM INFECTIOUS DISEASES STEWARDS

- Find allies in the surgical specialties, use them as messengers
- Learn about the intricacies and the needs of the unique surgical patient populations
- Understand how stressful diagnostic uncertainty can be in surgery
- Recognize the limits and morbidity of surgical treatment compared with medical management and be prepared to thoughtfully discuss

FROM SURGEONS, WHAT WE TELL OUR SURGICAL COLLEAGUES (AS ADVOCATES FOR STEWARDSHIP)

Having spent years working with outstanding antimicrobial stewardship teams, from time to time we are asked by surgeons how to make the relationship better. These are some tips for surgeons to help things run smoothly.

- Regarding prophylaxis, go to the meetings where protocols are designed and be involved with the decisions
- Once prophylaxis protocols are designed, stick to them

- Send cultures from the operating room where an infection is diagnosed, otherwise antimicrobial therapy is a shot in the dark. The lone exception may be community-acquired intra-abdominal infections
- With evolving technology, diagnosis is evolving. Accept changes suggested by the antimicrobial stewardship team, for example, diagnosis of *Clostridioides difficile* disease
- For empiric therapy of infections, choose a broad-spectrum regimen based on the disease condition and be consistent using it
- For complex, health care-associated infections, take the time to look up past clinical and colonization cultures and decide if empiric therapy should be altered
- Every time therapeutic antimicrobials are started, consider the end point, whether that is, based on days or response to therapy
- If a patient is deteriorating on antimicrobials, the first inclination should be to work on diagnostic considerations rather than adding more antimicrobials
- Take the time to communicate directly with members of the antimicrobial stewardship team, not just through notes, if you do not agree with their suggestions

HOW THE ANTIMICROBIAL STEWARDSHIP TEAM CAN MOST EFFECTIVELY WORK WITH SURGEONS

There are many ways for an antimicrobial stewardship team to build trust with surgeons. Some are given below.

- Include a personable pharmacist or physician on the team and use them to communicate in the acute setting
- Include at least 1 IDs expert who is willing to become expert in surgical infections and cultivate a trusting relationship with surgeons
- Openly acknowledge the expertise of the surgeon in terms of surgical management of complicated infections
- Demonstrate that you have considered the patient as a whole, not just an IDs problem
- Understand that the surgeons feel the greatest stress with decompensating patients without a clear diagnosis. Be flexible regarding the approval of antimicrobials while advocating for finding an infection source
- If disagreements are occurring consistently, sit down and compromise on a protocol or guidelines that all parties can accept based on data from literature as well as local issues and outcomes
- Find a surgeon that other surgeons trust, and when necessary, communicate through them, especially regarding policies
- Be willing to yield on small disagreements where interventions are probably equivalent
- Acknowledge when there are weak or nonexistent data to support your decisions
- Provide data for recommendations, and if possible, from the *surgical literature*, which may be more convincing to surgeons as it will more likely be done with more familiar approaches and outcomes
- Determine whether you want to devote your resources to preprescription authorization or postprescription review with feedback, although both are important. Surgeons far and away prefer the latter to the former, and literature supports that approach[12]
- Be the experts in diagnosis, especially with the coming wave of nucleic acid-based technologies that will have a new set of performance characteristics

DISCLOSURE

The authors have nothing to disclose.

REFERENCES

1. Anesi JA, Blumberg EA, Han JH, et al. Risk factors for multidrug-resistant organisms among deceased organ donors. Am J Transplant 2019;19(9): 2468–78.
2. Cardoso T, Ribeiro O, Aragao IC, et al. Additional risk factors for infection by multidrug-resistant pathogens in healthcare-associated infection: a large cohort study. BMC Infect Dis 2012;12:375.
3. Nseir S, Di Pompeo C, Soubrier S, et al. First-generation fluoroquinolone use and subsequent emergence of multiple drug-resistant bacteria in the intensive care unit. Crit Care Med 2005;33(2):283–9.
4. Safdar N, Maki DG. The commonality of risk factors for nosocomial colonization and infection with antimicrobial-resistant Staphylococcus aureus, enterococcus, gram-negative bacilli, Clostridium difficile, and Candida. Ann Intern Med 2002; 136(11):834–44.
5. Leeds IL, Fabrizio A, Cosgrove SE, et al. Treating wisely: the surgeon's role in antibiotic stewardship. Ann Surg 2017;265(5):871–3.
6. Tamma PD, Cosgrove SE. Antimicrobial stewardship. Infect Dis Clin North Am 2011;25(1):245–60.
7. Dortch MJ, Fleming SB, Kauffmann RM, et al. Infection reduction strategies including antibiotic stewardship protocols in surgical and trauma intensive care units are associated with reduced resistant gram-negative healthcare-associated infections. Surg Infect (Larchmt) 2011;12(1):15–25.
8. Barlam TF, Cosgrove SE, Abbo LM, et al. Implementing an antibiotic stewardship program: guidelines by the Infectious Diseases Society of America and the Society for Healthcare Epidemiology of America. Clin Infect Dis 2016; 62(10):e51–77.
9. Campbell KA, Stein S, Looze C, et al. Antibiotic stewardship in orthopaedic surgery: principles and practice. J Am Acad Orthop Surg 2014;22(12): 772–81.
10. Mehta JM, Haynes K, Wileyto EP, et al. Comparison of prior authorization and prospective audit with feedback for antimicrobial stewardship. Infect Control Hosp Epidemiol 2014;35(9):1092–9.
11. Sartelli M, Labricciosa FM, Scoccia L, et al. Non-restrictive antimicrobial stewardship program in a general and emergency surgery unit. Surg Infect (Larchmt) 2016;17(4):485–90.
12. Tamma PD, Avdic E, Keenan JF, et al. What is the more effective antibiotic stewardship intervention: preprescription authorization or postprescription review with feedback? Clin Infect Dis 2017;64(5):537–43.
13. Carling P, Fung T, Killion A, et al. Favorable impact of a multidisciplinary antibiotic management program conducted during 7 years. Infect Control Hosp Epidemiol 2003;24(9):699–706.
14. Libertin CR, Watson SH, Tillett WL, et al. Dramatic effects of a new antimicrobial stewardship program in a rural community hospital. Am J Infect Control 2017; 45(9):979–82.
15. Ruttimann S, Keck B, Hartmeier C, et al. Long-term antibiotic cost savings from a comprehensive intervention program in a medical department of a university-affiliated teaching hospital. Clin Infect Dis 2004;38(3):348–56.

16. Duane TM, Zuo JX, Wolfe LG, et al. Surgeons do not listen: evaluation of compliance with antimicrobial stewardship program recommendations. Am Surg 2013; 79(12):1269–72.
17. Sartelli M, Duane TM, Catena F, et al. Antimicrobial stewardship: a call to action for surgeons. Surg Infect (Larchmt) 2016;17(6):625–31.
18. Cakmakci M. Antibiotic stewardship programmes and the surgeon's role. J Hosp Infect 2015;89(4):264–6.
19. Munday GS, Deveaux P, Roberts H, et al. Impact of implementation of the Surgical Care Improvement Project and future strategies for improving quality in surgery. Am J Surg 2014;208(5):835–40.
20. Hennessy SA, Shah PM, Guidry CA, et al. Can nasal methicillin-resistant *Staphylococcus aureus* screening be used to avoid empiric vancomycin use in intra-abdominal infection? Surg Infect (Larchmt) 2015;16(4):396–400.
21. Paskovaty A, Pflomm JM, Myke N, et al. A multidisciplinary approach to antimicrobial stewardship: evolution into the 21st century. Int J Antimicrob Agents 2005;25(1):1–10.
22. Cairns KA, Bortz HD, Le A, et al. ICU antimicrobial stewardship (AMS) rounds: the daily activities of an AMS service. Int J Antimicrob Agents 2016;48(5):575–6.
23. Day SR, Smith D, Harris K, et al. An infectious diseases physician-led antimicrobial stewardship program at a small community hospital associated with improved susceptibility patterns and cost-savings after the first year. Open Forum Infect Dis 2015;2(2):ofv064.
24. Mclaughlin WL, Bowler JP, Holyoke JB. The causes of death following transurethral resection of the prostate. J Urol 1948;59(6):1233–42.
25. Davey P, Marwick CA, Scott CL, et al. Interventions to improve antibiotic prescribing practices for hospital inpatients. Cochrane Database Syst Rev 2017;(2):CD003543.
26. Feazel LM, Malhotra A, Perencevich EN, et al. Effect of antibiotic stewardship programmes on *Clostridium difficile* incidence: a systematic review and meta-analysis. J Antimicrob Chemother 2014;69(7):1748–54.
27. Ansari F, Erntell M, Goossens H, et al. The European surveillance of antimicrobial consumption (ESAC) point-prevalence survey of antibacterial use in 20 European hospitals in 2006. Clin Infect Dis 2009;49(10):1496–504.
28. Berríos-Torres SI, Umscheid CA, Bratzler DW, et al. Centers for disease control and prevention guideline for the prevention of surgical site infection, 2017. JAMA Surg 2017;152(8):784–91.
29. Branch-Elliman W, O'Brien W, Strymish J, et al. Association of duration and type of surgical prophylaxis with antimicrobial-associated adverse events. JAMA Surg 2019;154(7):590–8.
30. Oppelaar MC, Zijtveld C, Kuipers S, et al. Evaluation of prolonged vs short courses of antibiotic prophylaxis following ear, nose, throat, and oral and maxillofacial surgery: a systematic review and meta-analysis. JAMA Otolaryngol Head Neck Surg 2019;145(7):610–6.
31. Goede WJ, Lovely JK, Thompson RL, et al. Assessment of prophylactic antibiotic use in patients with surgical site infections. Hosp Pharm 2013;48(7):560–7.
32. Khaw C, Oberle AD, Lund BC, et al. Assessment of guideline discordance with antimicrobial prophylaxis best practices for common urologic procedures. JAMA Netw Open 2018;1(8):e186248.
33. Gandra S, Trett A, Alvarez-Uria G, et al. Is the efficacy of antibiotic prophylaxis for surgical procedures decreasing? Systematic review and meta-analysis of randomized control trials. Infect Control Hosp Epidemiol 2019;40(2):133–41.

34. Krebs ED, Hassinger TE, Guidry CA, et al. Non-utility of sepsis scores for identifying infection in surgical intensive care unit patients. Am J Surg 2019;218(2): 243–7.
35. Grill E, Weber A, Lohmann S, et al. Effects of pharmaceutical counselling on antimicrobial use in surgical wards: intervention study with historical control group. Pharmacoepidemiol Drug Saf 2011;20(7):739–46.

Collaborative Antimicrobial Stewardship in the Emergency Department

Nicole M. Acquisto, PharmD[a,b,*], Larissa May, MD, MSPH, MSHS[c]

KEYWORDS

- Antibiotic stewardship • Antimicrobial stewardship • Collaboration
- Emergency medicine • Emergency department

KEY POINTS

- The emergency department (ED) is an important clinical area to target for antimicrobial stewardship (AS) efforts based on high rates of antibiotic overprescribing and antimicrobial adverse event–related ED visits.
- Patient information and microbiologic data often are lacking, and high patient volumes, frequent interruptions, large diversity of patients, and pressures for throughput, coupled with concerns about patient follow-up and satisfaction, make ED AS efforts challenging.
- The ED is positioned between ambulatory and inpatient care, making AS collaborations between the institution and community important for success.
- ED AS efforts should focus on avoidance of unnecessary antibiotics; selection of the right drug, dose, and duration; appropriate diagnostic tests; prompt administration; and preventing ED return/readmission.
- Future acute-care AS initiatives could focus on health care system expansion, targeting pediatrics and urgent care settings, and routine follow-up for antibiotic de-escalation.

INTRODUCTION AND IMPORTANCE TO THE EMERGENCY DEPARTMENT

Inappropriate antimicrobial use leading to antibiotic resistance is a major public health concern. Antibiotic stewardship (AS) defined as "coordinated interventions designed to improve and measure the appropriate use of [antibiotic] agents by promoting the selection of optimal [antibiotic] drug regimen including, dosing, duration of therapy, and route of administration" are necessary to mitigate antimicrobial resistance and reduce antibiotic-related adverse events.[1,2]

[a] Department of Pharmacy, University of Rochester Medical Center, 601 Elmwood Avenue, Box 638, Rochester, NY 14642, USA; [b] Department of Emergency Medicine, University of Rochester Medical Center, 601 Elmwood Avenue, Box 655, Rochester, NY 14642, USA; [c] Department of Emergency Medicine, University of California, Davis Health, 4150 V Street Patient Support Services Building (PSSB), Suite 2100, Sacramento, CA 95817, USA
* Corresponding author. 601 Elmwood Avenue, Box 638, Rochester, NY 14642,
E-mail address: nicole_acquisto@urmc.rochester.edu
Twitter: @nacquisto (N.M.A.); @LSMayMD (L.M.)

Infect Dis Clin N Am 34 (2020) 109–127
https://doi.org/10.1016/j.idc.2019.10.004
0891-5520/20/© 2019 Elsevier Inc. All rights reserved.

Although management of high-acuity patients is foundational to emergency medicine (EM) practice, most patients evaluated in the emergency department (ED) are discharged to home or a long-term care facility (LTCF). Of the 145 million ED visits reported in 2016, only 10% were admitted to the hospital.[3] Of the top 10 reasons for ED visits, 7 in the pediatric and 4 in the adult population may be related to an infectious disease (pediatrics: fever, cough, stomach/abdominal pain, vomiting, skin rash, symptoms referable to throat, and earache/ear infection; adults: stomach/abdominal pain, symptoms referable to throat, cough, and shortness of breath). Importantly, of 117 million medication mentions, antibiotics account for 29 million, or 25%, making it the fourth largest therapeutic drug class used in the ED after analgesics, antiemetics, and minerals/electrolytes.[3] Although improvements in antibiotic prescribing have been made, it is still reported that 30% to 50% of outpatient prescriptions are unnecessary or inappropriate based on antibiotic selection, dose, and duration.[4–11] Specifically, unnecessary antibiotics are prescribed in 32 to 74% of pediatric and adult patients for common viral respiratory infections (acute bronchitis, bronchiolitis, upper respiratory infection -[URI]) and in 25% for SSTI, resulting in millions of unnecessary antibiotic courses.[10–13]

Aside from the impact on antimicrobial resistance, there is a direct effect on the number of ED visits and hospital admissions for adverse drug events related to antimicrobials. In 2013 to 2014, 16% of all medication-related adverse events in adults presenting to the ED involved antimicrobials.[14] Allergic reactions were the most common (82%; 18% severe), followed by gastrointestinal, sensory/motor disturbances, neurologic, and secondary infections including, candidiasis and *Clostridioides difficile*. Among children 5 years old and younger (includes 5 yo) and those 6 years old to 19 years old, antibiotics alone were implicated in 56% and 32% of ED visits for adverse drug events, respectively, and resulted in hospitalization in 27%.[14] This has a direct impact in driving up ED utilization and contributes to unnecessary direct health care and societal costs.

CHALLENGES OF ANTIMICROBIAL STEWARDSHIP IN THE EMERGENCY DEPARTMENT

The ED is a unique practice site where clinicians are positioned between the community and acute-care setting.[4] Improving AS practices in the ED is not a simple solution. The ED environment itself is challenging because there is a high volume of patients in an often overcrowded setting. There are pressures for patient throughput, frequent interruptions, and a diverse population with pediatric, adult, and geriatric patients, with low-acuity to high-acuity disease states being managed simultaneously. There are many obstacles for ED clinicians, including limited time to spend with each patient, rapid patient turnover, lack of continuity of care, concerns with patient satisfaction, medical liability for failure to diagnose or treat, and pressures to meet Centers for Medicare and Medicaid Services Core Quality Measures while at the same time needing to be thoughtful about appropriate antibiotic prescribing and overuse.[15–18] Furthermore, there is not a uniform model of emergency care. In most settings, EM physicians and other clinicians do not work directly for the health care system they practice in but work for contracted groups or are independent contractors working in multiple settings. These obstacles are occurring in a high-pressure setting where it often is difficult to obtain thorough patient information, such as history of present illness, historical antibiotic use, or outside sources of microbiologic results. Patients in the ED also present with the full spectrum of illness severity, ranging from minor viral infections to life-threatening sepsis, leading to the need to balance potentially inappropriate empiric antibiotic selection in the setting of limited diagnostic information and urgency of presentation. For the antimicrobial steward, there are even more challenges due to high EM clinician turnover rates, dissimilar clinical commitments, and differences in practices, experience, and knowledge related to appropriate antibiotic use among individual clinicians.

Given EM clinicians are high prescribers of antimicrobials and the many challenges related to practicing in the ED environment, the ED and urgent care settings have been targeted for the development of antimicrobial stewardship programs (ASPs) in recent years.[19-23] The Centers for Disease Control and Prevention (CDC) Core Elements of Outpatient Antibiotic Stewardship, which provides a framework for AS in the outpatient setting, is intended for use in ED and urgent care settings and the Infectious Diseases Society of America (IDSA) and the Society for Healthcare Epidemiology (SHEA) guidelines on Implementing an Antimicrobial Stewardship Program recommend expansion of AS activities to the ED.[2,4]

ESTABLISHING A COLLABORATIVE ANTIMICROBIAL STEWARDSHIP PROGRAM TEAM

Building a leadership infrastructure is important to the success of an ED ASP. First, identification of a program champion (physician, pharmacist, or other health care professional) to lead education, communicate initiatives, organize collaborations, promote stewardship activities, and disseminate data follow-up and feedback is necessary.[22,23] Collaboration is the foundation for an effective ASP because it is complex and multifaceted (**Table 1**). This issue details the importance of collaborators and the ED is no exception. There is no department quite like the ED when describing collaborative practice teams. The ED touches almost every department and division in an institution and beyond, with a diverse patient population and varying patient dispositions. When considering key collaborators, it is important to consider not only the EM team (departmental director, nursing leadership, clinicians, nurses, and pharmacists) but also ambulatory or primary care providers, LTCFs, admitting medical teams, and outpatient pharmacies. Other collaborators within the institution should be considered: infectious diseases (ID) colleagues, clinical microbiologists, hospital epidemiologists and infection prevention programs, information technology (IT) services, and quality improvement professionals.[23] Hospital leadership sponsorship and a program manager are key members to obtain and maintain success.[23] Most hospitals have already existing ASPs, but to engage other health care professionals, create an understanding of existing barriers in the ED and workflow, and engage front-line ED clinicians in AS it is important to have ED-specific representation on these committees.[19]

An EM pharmacist should be considered a strategic partner. Clinical pharmacists as collaborators and leaders in ASPs is supported by the IDSA/SHEA guidelines and the Society of Infectious Diseases Pharmacists.[1,2,24] EM pharmacists play a crucial role in appropriate antimicrobial selection at the bedside and provide real-time consultation, education, and feedback to clinicians.[19,20,22,25] They have an astute understanding of provider prescribing practices, ED workflow, and relevant outcome measures and can develop, lead, assist, and promote ASP initiatives.[21,25-40] A multicenter evaluation of medication errors intercepted by EM pharmacists found that pharmacist consultation compared with order review yielded more interceptions, 51% versus 35%, supporting pharmacists practicing physically in the ED.[41] Most errors were related to wrong dose (44%) or wrong drug (14%); 40% of medication error interceptions were antibiotic related (unpublished data). Other studies have found that pharmacists involved in direct patient care activities in the ED improves guideline-concordant antibiotic

Table 1
Emergency department antimicrobial stewardship strategies and suggested collaborations

Strategies	Relevant Partners[a]
Empiric antimicrobial treatment—right drug, dose, duration	
ED-specific guidelines	EM clinicians, EM pharmacists, infectious disease clinicians, ambulatory clinicians, LTCF clinicians
ED antibiogram	Microbiology
Guideline implementation	IT services, EM pharmacists
Behavioral economics and nudging	EM clinicians, EM pharmacists, quality improvement professionals, IT services
Rapid diagnostic testing	Microbiology, EM clinicians, EM nurses, ambulatory clinicians
Medication availability	EM pharmacist/pharmacy department
Discharge prescription review	IT services, EM clinicians, EM pharmacists
Prompt administration	
Sepsis initiatives	EM clinicians, critical care clinicians, EM pharmacists, EM nurses, quality improvement professionals, IT services
Streamline administration	EM pharmacist/pharmacy department, EM clinicians, specialty service clinicians,[b] EM nurses, IT services
Prevent ED return/readmissions	
Culture surveillance and follow-up	EM pharmacists, EM clinicians, infectious disease clinicians, ambulatory clinicians, LTCF clinicians, hospital epidemiologists and infection control professionals or colleagues
Take-home medication packs	EM clinicians, infectious disease clinicians, EM pharmacists/pharmacy department
Blood cultures	EM clinicians, EM nurses, infectious disease clinicians, microbiology, IT services
Future initiatives	
Telephone follow-up	Care coordinators, EM nurses, EM pharmacists, quality improvement representative
Antibiotic de-escalation	EM clinicians, EM pharmacists, ambulatory clinicians, outpatient pharmacy
Antibiotic cessation	EM clinicians, EM pharmacists, ambulatory clinicians, outpatient pharmacy
Target pediatrics	EM clinicians, pediatric EM clinicians, infectious disease clinicians, pediatric infectious disease clinicians, pediatric clinicians, EM pharmacists
Target urgent care centers	EM clinicians, EM pharmacists, local public health representatives, health insurance companies
Telemedicine/telehealth	EM clinicians, EM pharmacists, services

[a] All partnerships described would be in collaboration with emergency department AS program leadership.
[b] Oncologists, Orthopedists, or Traumatologists.

prescribing and appropriate dosing compared with when a pharmacist is not present.[26,28–32]

Education is an important component of an effective ED ASP and each individual AS intervention. The ASP team must collaborate with ED thought leaders to tailor education for optimal engagement.[19] Education alone, however, is not likely to lead to sustained change. Multifaceted education with audit and feedback, 1-on-1 instruction, and peer comparisons has been shown to be effective for AS in targeted disease states.[21] Along with a clinician champion and other members of the ED AS team, an EM pharmacist is uniquely positioned to provide continuous education and feedback. Education can occur at different points in the prescribing process: proactively through consultation with the EM pharmacist, active feedback in response to a medication order, or retrospectively from culture surveillance and follow-up activities.[20] Ultimately, EM pharmacist participation in different ED ASPs can optimize antimicrobial use, improve guideline-concordant selection and dose, reduce time to medication administration in life-threatening infections, reduce medication errors, improve transitions of care, and decrease readmissions.[21,25–40]

Recently the American Nurses Association partnered with the CDC to facilitate engagement of nurses in AS activities, identify gaps to participation in initiatives, and explore opportunities for an expanded role.[42] Nurses often are the epicenter of patient care and communication with the health care team and work closest with patients and their families in the hospital, community, and at home. This puts them in a unique position to educate patients and families and advocate for appropriate antimicrobial use. In the ED, nurses spend considerably more 1-on-1 time with the patient during the ED visit and often are responsible for appropriate patient triage, accurate allergy history, obtaining early and appropriate cultures, timely antibiotic administration, discharge plan and prescription review with the patient, and communication with the inpatient unit or LTCFs at ED discharge. In some models, the nurse is responsible for obtaining medication histories and completing culture surveillance and follow-up. Therefore, it is important to engage nurses in ED AS efforts and have nursing leadership as a key partner aligned with the ED ASP champion.

STRATEGIES FOR ANTIMICROBIAL STEWARDSHIP IN THE EMERGENCY DEPARTMENT

The ED is unique for stewardship in that patients are often in the department for only a short period of time. Some traditional AS activities like preauthorization, de-escalation of therapy, intravenous (IV) to oral interchange, and scheduled antimicrobial evaluation at 48 hours or 72 hours may not be conducive to ED care. EM clinicians have the additional challenge of routinely working with 2 different patient dispositions; those being discharged (approximately 90%, to home or to another health care facility like an LTCF) or admitted (approximately 10%), depending on the setting. Furthermore, managing patients with severe infections that warrant appropriate initial broad-spectrum antibiotics but also deciphering between viral and bacterial infections and selecting appropriate empiric, narrow spectrum, or no antibiotic treatment can be challenging. Again, because the ED is responsible for an important but limited piece of patient care, collaboration with the rest of the health care team in the community and hospital is necessitated for optimal stewardship strategies. It is important to recognize that antimicrobial decisions made in the ED influence outpatient and inpatient care; when guideline-concordant prescribing occurred in the ED, appropriate therapy was continued on admission compared with when inappropriate therapy was started in the ED for pneumonia and intra-abdominal infections (83% vs 19%).[31]

The CDC Core Elements of Outpatient Antibiotic Stewardship recommend focusing on 1 or more high-priority conditions for intervention, conditions where (1) antibiotics are overprescribed (eg, acute sinusitis, acute uncomplicated bronchitis, upper respiratory tract infection, viral pharyngitis, acute otitis media, bronchiolitis, and asymptomatic bacteriuria); (2) antibiotics may be appropriate but conditions are over-diagnosed (eg, streptococcal pharyngitis without positive testing); (3) antibiotics are indicated but wrong drug, dose, or duration; (4) watchful waiting/delayed prescribing (symptomatic relief and antibiotic contingency plan if symptoms do not improve or worsen); or (5) antibiotics are underused or not timely (eg, sepsis).[4]

There are several strategies to target these high-priority AS conditions in the ED, which can be categorized into 3 main areas:

1. Empiric antimicrobial treatment: decision to treat and selection of right drug, dose, and duration
2. Prompt antimicrobial administration
3. Prevent ED returns/readmissions

Empiric Antimicrobial Treatment

Emergency department–specific guidelines

Local clinical practice guidelines frequently are adapted from national guidelines and focus on appropriate indications for antimicrobials in addition to providing recommendations for medication selection, dose, and duration. There are several important points to consider that necessitate ED-specific adaptation or development of separate materials. First, the ED antimicrobial formulary compared with the inpatient formulary must be considered. Second, guidance must also include when *not* to treat with antimicrobials. Third, inpatient guidelines are developed using inpatient susceptibilities or the summation of ED and inpatient susceptibilities and may overestimate resistance patterns, resulting in exclusion of antimicrobials with more narrow spectrum coverage. Reports comparing ED and inpatient isolates found significant differences showing greater antimicrobial susceptibilities of ED isolates.[43,44] Furthermore, 1 report evaluated group-specific urinary antibiograms of patients from the community versus an LTCF and in different age groups (greater than or less than 50 years old and 65 years old) and found distinct differences.[45] There is still a risk that an ED-specific antibiogram overestimates local resistance because there is bias to obtaining microbiologic culture for sicker patients or those with comorbidities. Nonetheless, collaborating with clinical microbiology colleagues to develop an ED-specific antibiogram can help preserve the use of some antimicrobials and should be used for ED clinical practice guidelines development or adaptation.[21]

Antimicrobial overprescribing is a significant problem in the ED, and there is much attention to address appropriate prescribing for acute respiratory infections, urinary tract infections (UTIs), and SSTIs.[22,23] Developing recommendations for both when and when *not* to test and when and when *not* to treat must be collaborative, because patient care will be transitioned to ambulatory or inpatient clinicians. Without collaboration and ensuring there is agreement among clinicians, ED AS interventions may be futile. For instance, during a UTI work-up, there are external factors to consider related to the decision to obtain a urine culture, culture interpretation, and UTI diagnosis. The choice to obtain a urinary culture could have an impact on the patient at other points of care because ambulatory or inpatient clinicians may inherit these results. For example, an elderly patient presents with confusion, odorous urine, and a recent fall. An EM clinician following ED urine culture criteria developed with infectious disease, hospital medicine, long-term care, and ambulatory colleagues, decides not to obtain a culture, recognizing that screening and/or treatment of asymptomatic bacteriuria is not recommended in most patient populations.[46] The patient's confusion resolves with hydration and they are discharged. Alternate scenarios may be that the patient also reported a fever and was hypotensive and the EM clinician obtains a urinalysis with reflex to culture and (1) empirically treats; (2) is obliged to treat because the LTCF, without a robust ASP, requires treatment for the patient to return; or (3) decides not to treat based on ED improvement. The urine culture is now on a consequential path where it may be evaluated during ED culture surveillance and follow-up activities or by ambulatory, LTCF, or inpatient clinicians, all with the potential to change the antibiotic regimen based on susceptibilities or initiate antibiotic treatment.

It is important for EM clinicians to thoughtfully consider microbiologic culture and avoid any potential negative downstream consequences by ensuring the rationale and plan are clearly documented and communicated during care transition. On the other hand, clinical evaluation and de-escalation of therapy is a common approach to inpatient AS. When appropriate, it is important for EM clinicians to obtain relevant cultures before antibiotics are initiated for the inpatient team to have organism identification and susceptibility information to guide care decisions.[19] Both of these scenarios demonstrate the importance of collaboration and communication throughout transitions of care and a requisite understanding of ED-specific guidelines and workflows.

Guideline Implementation
Guidelines often are developed based on individual disease states, may have different outlined clinical pathways based on patent-specific clinical factors (eg, purulent or no purulent drainage with SSTI) and can be lengthy. Operationalizing guidelines in the electronic medical record (EMR)/physician order entry systems, through collaboration with IT colleagues, can support appropriate clinical treatment pathways and deter inappropriate prescribing. These tools can be developed at the presumed diagnosis or medication level to guide clinicians to appropriate antibiotic therapy or nudge clinicians to suggested nonantibiotic alternatives.[47,48] One report describes a clinical decision support tool initiated at the medication level, azithromycin or gatifloxacin, followed by selection of respiratory diagnosis and clinical criteria that reduced unnecessary prescriptions from 22% to 3%.[47] Similarly, a pop-up, triggered by certain acute respiratory tract infection diagnoses, suggesting that antibiotics are not indicated and providing a list of alternative symptomatic treatments that could be ordered, reduced mean antibiotic prescribing rates by 16%.[48]

Other electronic tools like antibiotic order forms or order sets with the appropriate medication or combination of medications, frequency, and duration defaulted, may help direct prescribing practices. Importantly in the ED, these can be built for ED and inpatient use but also for discharge prescription generation. Accountable justification through an EMR prompt is another behavioral intervention to consider. This requires the clinician to include written justification for antimicrobial use that is documented in the medication record for both antibiotic appropriate and inappropriate diagnoses. Incorporating accountability can improve the quality of decision making, can reduce antibiotic prescribing rates, and is valuable for surveillance and identification of future AS target areas for optimization.[49] Alternatively, it is important to review already existing models and previously built clinical decision support or order sets to identify any contributing factors to antibiotic overuse, such as unnecessary or inappropriate antimicrobial regimens or microbiologic cultures (eg, urine or blood). For example, collaborative practices that leverage the EMR and clinical decision support can help reduce inappropriate treatment of asymptomatic bacteriuria by reducing the number of inappropriate urine cultures sent from the ED.[49,50] Routine review of any of these electronic tools should be coordinated with the ED ASP champion and IT services.

Behavioral economics and nudging

Recognizing that the ED is a complex environment where clinicians are bound by heuristics and where decisions frequently are subconscious and impacted by multiple psychosocial and environmental factors, there is an opportunity for the use of nudges, or gentle persuaders, that steer clinicians to avoidance of unnecessary antibiotics, through the use of peer comparisons, accountable justification (described previously), and the concept of public commitment statements and posters pledging to avoid patient harm from unneeded antibiotics.

A recent multicenter randomized controlled trial of 9 ED and urgent care sites in 3 different health care systems, the MITIGATE trial, compared the effectiveness of an antibiotic stewardship intervention to reduce inappropriate prescribing for viral respiratory infections adapted for acute-care ambulatory settings (adapted intervention—education for patients and clinicians and general department feedback) to a stewardship intervention (enhanced intervention—education in addition to individualized audit and feedback, peer comparisons, and behavioral nudges) in reducing inappropriate prescription.[51] Antibiotic prescribing for acute respiratory infection visits dropped from 2.2% (95% CI, 1.0% to 3.4%) to 1.5% (95% CI, 0.7% to 2.3%) with an odds ratio of 0.67 (95% CI, 0.54–0.82). Difference-in-differences between the 2 interventions were not significantly different likely due to low rates of inappropriate prescribing at baseline in these academic centers. This study used an implementation science approach, which provides a conceptual framework to more rigorously and effectively translate evidence-based interventions into practice.

Rapid diagnostic testing

Microbiological data from culture growth, identification, and susceptibility testing are delayed several days and unavailable during clinical decision making in the ED. Rapid diagnostic testing and point-of-care and rapid molecular tests along with clinical risk assessment have the potential to assist with decisions to treat or not with antimicrobials, allow more narrow-spectrum empiric regimens, and assist with disposition decision.[22] Rapid streptococcal testing lowered antibiotic prescribing rate from 41% to 23% in a sample of more than 8000 patients from 1 pediatric ED (false-negative results, 0.04%).[52] Similarly, rapid influenza assays have assisted with diagnosis, reduced ED antimicrobial use (23% vs 11%), and increased antiviral use.[53] A limitation of these polymerase chain reaction assays is that they only test for a single viral etiology. Rapid multiplex respiratory viral panels, that test up to 20 common pathogens, are now available; however, regardless of positive or negative result, they did not show a difference in antibiotic prescribing for noninfluenza viruses in an evaluation of ED and urgent care patients.[54] Compared with traditional testing, individual rapid influenza and respiratory syncytial virus tests produce a more rapid turnaround time for result but these have not been associated with reduced overall ED treatment time.[55,56] Importantly, though, more patients have test results before ED discharge and fewer blood culture, blood gas, sputum culture, and respiratory bacterial and viral serology tests were ordered for patients tested by rapid influenza and respiratory syncytial virus PCR in an Australian ED.[56] These mixed results suggest an opportunity for AS guidance of diagnostic test implementation and management.

Many clinicians use risk assessment and evidence of purulence to guide antibiotic prescribing for SSTIs, but this can result in routine double antibiotic coverage or a regimen with higher risk of antibiotic-related adverse effects than necessary.[21] A report in 1 ED found that treatment concordant with guideline recommendations was low in patients presenting with SSTIs; unnecessary or nonrecommended antibiotics were started in approximately 70% of patients, each with nonpurulent or purulent infections and mild abscesses were almost always treated with antibiotics.[57] Methicillin-resistant Staphylococcus aureus (MRSA) nares carriage and rapid molecular MRSA testing have been investigated as tools to tailor antibiotic therapy for patients with SSTIs presenting to the ED. MRSA nares carriage was found to be a better predictor of MRSA wound infection compared with clinical risk factors alone.[58] Those who tested positive for either methicillin-sensitive Staphylococcus aureus or MRSA when using rapid molecular testing received targeted antibiotics, although there were no differences in overall antibiotic use.[59] These can be important tools to consider to reduce overall antibiotic exposure (1 vs 2 empiric antibiotics) in patients with SSTIs.

Patients routinely present to the ED for evaluation and treatment of sexually transmitted infections. Routine empiric treatment to prevent transmission spread is standard practice but associated with antibiotic overuse and growing resistance.[21] Nucleic acid amplification tests used in the ED for chlamydia and gonorrhea with real-time reporting have decreased unnecessary antibiotics in those testing negative and increased adherence to antibiotics.[60,61] With these benefits and improved notification of positive testing results compared with batch testing, 75% of clinicians felt that a 90-minute turnaround time for rapid testing disrupted their workflow.[61] The future availability of US Food and Drug Administration–waived rapid tests for gonorrhea and chlamydia under the Clinical Laboratory Improvement Amendments has the potential to be integrated into clinical workflow and lead to improved patient management and follow-up.[62]

Detecting procalcitonin (PCT), a biomarker up-regulated during bacterial infection, may help differentiate bacterial versus viral infection. A multicenter study performed in 6 EDs in Switzerland randomized patients with a primary diagnosis of lower respiratory tract infection (eg, community-acquired pneumonia, chronic obstructive pulmonary disease, or bronchitis) to PCT algorithm or evidence-based guidelines for care. Their finding suggest lower antibiotic prescribing (75% vs 88%), less antibiotic exposure (5.7 vs 8.7 days), and reduced antibiotic adverse events (19% vs 28%) without a difference in overall adverse outcomes when the PCT algorithm is incorporated into clinical decision.[63] Implementation and integration of PCT into the clinical workflow and AS procedures is an important consideration for future evaluation. A recent multicenter ED-based randomized controlled trial of a PCT protocol versus usual care found no significant difference in antibiotic days between 2 groups (4.2 days and 4.3 days); this was possibly due to lack of familiarity or experience with PCT, challenges with assay interpretation, and the wrong targeted population (patients being admitted to the hospital with pneumonia).[64]

Collaboration between clinical microbiology colleagues and the ED is necessary for rapid diagnostic testing success. False-positive and false-negative rates, laboratory workflow constraints, turnaround time, and cost should be understood by EM clinicians and minimized, when possible, to improve the utility of these tests in the ED. It is necessary to determine logistical and potential regulatory issues before widespread use and if any individual test should be restricted to certain populations (eg, respiratory viral panel for immunocompromised patients only). Obtaining a PCT may have an impact on the ED decision to initiate antibiotics, but ambulatory and inpatient clinicians must understand how to use the algorithm and when clinical reevaluation and PCT measurement should occur. This highlights the need for collaboration and communication across all patient transitions when biomarkers are used in the ED.

Medication availability

There are many opportunities to collaborate with a pharmacy department to optimize medication availability in the ED. This can help drive appropriate prescribing practices and ensure prompt administration. It has been shown that moving medications to an ED automated dispensing cabinet from a central hospital pharmacy can increase the frequency of prescribing.[65] Ensuring that preferred antibiotics for common infections recommended in EDs and institutional guidelines and used in order sets are readily available, whereas restricted and nonformulary medications are not, will assist *appropriate* prescribing. Clinicians also can be directed to use these products through annotations next to product names in the EMR or the use of an ED-specific preference list. Annotations also can alert clinicians to antibiotic products that are readily available in certain medical dispensing cabinets in the ED (eg, antibiotics noted with "Peds" may be in a specific pediatric ED medication dispensing cabinet or a preferred product for that patient population). Pharmacy batching of certain medication strengths, such as vancomycin, 1500 mg or 2000 mg, to ensure a consistent supply is readily available in the ED medication dispensing cabinets can influence appropriate dose prescribing and improve time to antibiotic administration for those with life-threatening infections.

Prescription review

ED discharge prescription medication errors occur in approximately 23% of pediatric and 10% of adult prescriptions.[66,67] In 1 review of 1000 discharge prescriptions, errors occurred with antibiotic prescriptions more often than in any other class (17%).[66] Incomplete/inadequate prescriptions (58%), drug selection errors (22%), and dosing outside the recommended range (20%) occurred most often. This can result in suboptimal therapy, risk of adverse events, and potential gaps or delays in treatment. Also, fielding telephone calls from outpatient pharmacies if these errors are intercepted, often to a clinician who did not see the patient initially, adds interruptions and additional work to the already stressed ED workflow.

Prescription review by an EM pharmacist before discharge or electronic prescribing transmission is another strategy that could be used to ensure the right drug, dose, and duration. Although not specific to antibiotics, EM pharmacists intervened on 10% of discharge prescriptions (23.6% pediatrics and 8.5% adults) to prevent medication error (54%) or optimize therapy (46%) in 1 prospective, observational study.[67] More than 95% of clinicians surveyed believed this pharmacist service improved patient safety, optimized medication regimens, and improved patient satisfaction.[67] With electronic prescribing, it is important to engage IT colleagues, EM clinicians, and EM pharmacists to develop a discharge prescription process that it efficient, is collaborative, and does not inhibit patient throughput. This could be an optimal AS initiative for a physician-pharmacist collaborative practice agreement, in which a pharmacist could independently manage antibiotic changes under an agreed-on protocol. This should not circumvent direct feedback to clinicians regarding inappropriate antibiotic selection, dose, or duration.

Prompt Antimicrobial Administration

Sepsis

Appropriate, early administration of antibiotics improves outcomes in patients with severe sepsis/septic shock and is part of the Surviving Sepsis Campaign Hour-1 Bundle.[68] Collaboration with EM and critical care clinicians, EM pharmacists, nurses, and IT services is necessary to optimize patient screening for sepsis (or automate in the EMR using objective patient information) and ordering and administration of antibiotics to meet these goals. Pharmacists physically practicing in the ED can assist with guideline development, appropriate antibiotic selection, development of tools in the EMR to guide appropriate selection, medication availability in the ED, and prompt antibiotic administration in response to a sepsis alert, bedside consultation, or medication order. EM pharmacists as part of an ED sepsis alert team reduced time to appropriate antibiotics by a median 44 minutes.[28] Similarly, EM pharmacists physically in the ED improved the likelihood of receiving antibiotics within 1 hour (88% vs 72%) for sepsis/severe sepsis/septic shock patients compared with when a pharmacist was not present in the ED.[29] EM pharmacists also can provide bedside education to nurses on the order of antibiotic administration for limited IV access and multiple antibiotic orders, answer questions about allergies or rate of administration that could delay administration, and promote other aspects of the bundle like obtaining blood cultures and lactate concentration. Importantly, related to sepsis care after patient admission, it is imperative for EM clinicians to order appropriate cultures for critical care and other inpatient clinicians to have microbiologic data available to ensure appropriate antimicrobial coverage and allow de-escalation as necessary.

Streamline administration
Limited IV access, lack of medication infusion compatibility, and patients leaving the ED for extended periods of time for additional work-up all may affect timely antibiotic administration. Although sepsis often is a primary focus in the ED, rapid antibiotic administration for open fracture prophylaxis and febrile neutropenia have emerged as national recommendations and quality measures.[69–71] Rapid triage and diagnosis along with appropriate antibiotic ordering, ED medication availability, and prompt administration require collaboration with EM clinicians, specialty service providers, pharmacists, nurses, and IT services. One strategy to aid with administration issues and improve time to first dose is to develop a process for IV-push antibiotic administration instead of an IV infusion when available.[72] This requires collaboration with pharmacy and nursing to ensure the appropriate IV product is available and for overall education on the process change and rationale. Additionally, EM pharmacists participating in direct patient care activities during trauma resuscitation were associated with a higher proportion of patients receiving initial antibiotics in accordance with national recommendations (81% vs 47%) and more timely administration compared with when a pharmacist was not present in the ED.[32]

Febrile and neutropenic patients seen in the ED often are advised by their outpatient oncologist to present to the ED. A collaborative process where the oncologist can call ahead to the ED, the EM clinician can order antibiotics in the EMR, and preparation of antibiotics (may be from the central hospital pharmacy for pediatrics) can be started even before ED arrival may improve time to antibiotic administration. These processes require coordinated efforts and education to be successful.

Prevent Emergency Department Return/Readmissions

Culture surveillance and follow-up
Culture and susceptibility information often is not available for several days after patient discharge from the ED. Bug-drug match/mismatch, de-escalation, and the need to initiate/change antibiotics are easily evaluated by the inpatient team for admitted patients. It is necessary in the ED setting to develop a structured follow-up program to evaluate these data and provide appropriate follow-up for discharged patients (eg, changing or initiating antibiotics, contacting primary or specialty care offices or the department of health, or returning to the ED). Setting up this program requires collaboration with the ED, Department of Microbiology, IT services to build the routing pool, and ambulatory and LTCF clinicians who receive

results is necessary for success.[33] Microbiology, hospital epidemiology, and infection control colleagues can inform the process for state-reportable results and notification of positive sterile site cultures. EM pharmacist–managed programs in the ED have improved the time to culture review and physician notification, increased appropriate antibiotic interventions, reduced inappropriate interventions, reduced ED returns by approximately 12% in 2 separate studies, and saved EM clinician time.[34–38] Similarly, remote pharmacist–led culture follow-up for urgent cares have result in improved appropriate antibiotic interventions and guideline-concordant antibiotic prescribing.[39,40] Having the same group of health care professionals manage this program daily is advantageous to identify trends in prescribing to develop further AS initiatives, identify any gaps in culture or serology result routing, and create opportunities for direct feedback and education for clinicians. This type of pharmacist-physician collaboration creates an opportunity for formal collaborative practice agreement as well.

Take-home medication packs
Writing a discharge prescription does not ensure that a patient actually receives the medication. Medication nonadherence may occur due to cost, insurance coverage, transportation, and pharmacy hours (closed at ED discharge time). One investigation targeted patients with these presumed barriers to filling a discharge prescription and a diagnosis of UTI, pyelonephritis, cellulitis, or dental infection to receive a take-home medication pack of appropriate antibiotics (individualized dose and duration) at ED discharge.[73] At a nominal cost, $1123 for 243 take-home medication packs, ED returns within 7 days were reduced by more than 50% compared with patients who received a prescription at discharge (standard of care). Providing individualized medication packs at the correct dose and duration also influences appropriate prescribing practices. Another study that evaluated take-home medication packs for a wide variety of medications (11/20 were antibiotics but were not individualized to dose and duration based on indication) did not find a difference in 30-day ED returns.[74] Providing take-home medications for targeted disease states requires collaboration with EM clinicians, EM pharmacists, and infectious disease clinicians to determine a set formulary, dose, and duration and the pharmacy department for kit development and storage.

Blood cultures
Unnecessary blood cultures are obtained in the ED and may result in false-positive results, leading to needless clinical evaluation, additional communication with the patient or ambulatory care clinicians, unnecessary re-presentation to the ED or readmission to the hospital, additional laboratory tests, avoidable antibiotic exposure, and increased health care costs. AS strategies to reduce these occurrences involve collaboration with EM clinicians, nurses, infectious disease clinicians, and clinical microbiology colleagues. Key strategies are to prevent unnecessary blood culture sampling, reduce contamination rates, and improve blood culture evaluation to identify false-positive results compared with true-positive results.

In recent years, blood culture sampling for community-acquired pneumonia has been removed from Centers for Medicare and Medicaid Services Core Quality Measures due to limited utility of these having an impact on management decisions or leading to better outcomes and the risk of false-positive results influencing inappropriate antimicrobial use and length of hospital stay.[75] Removing routine blood culture orders from order sets where they are not necessary, using clinical decision support for ordering blood cultures, and collaborating with nursing to prevent preemptive drawing of blood cultures before orders are placed through education are additional possible strategies.

High rates of blood culture contamination contribute to downstream misused resources. Programs focused on improving ED blood culture sampling techniques and sterile procedures, specimen diversion devices, phlebotomist draw, or procedural checklists are an area for AS collaboration with ED nursing.[76–79] The Department of Microbiology can provide tracking of contaminated blood culture rates to evaluate ED interventions to reduce these rates.

Collaboration with clinical microbiology colleagues, EM clinicians, pharmacists, or nurses interpreting these cultures is necessary. To limit action on false-positive blood cultures, laboratory or clinical algorithms can be implemented.[80] Nucleic acid detection (Blood culture nucleic acid detection) or proteomic-based methods using mass spectrometry (matrix-assisted laser desorption/ionization time-of-flight) can provide rapid organism detection that is valuable for interpretation and determining appropriate follow-up or necessary patient reevaluation.[81,82] Collaborating with clinical microbiology colleagues to understand and optimize timing of pulling signal-positive bottles, when rapid molecular test is performed and turnaround time, and the process for alerting of a positive culture and reporting in the EMR is important to operationalize the clinical utility of these tests during blood culture evaluation.

FUTURE OF EMERGENCY DEPARTMENT ANTIMICROBIAL STEWARDSHIP

Although there have been several successful ED AS strategies described, the following gaps related to - patient follow-up after discharge, de-escalation of therapy, cessation of therapy after symptoms resolution, targeting pediatric and urgent care setting populations, and creating health care system-wide acute-care AS strategies—still need to be addressed.

Patients discharged from the ED and hospital often are contacted via telephone for transitions of care coordination, evaluation of satisfaction of care, and an opportunity for questions. These calls (and other novel communication techniques) could be used to educate patients about their infectious illness and antibiotic use, address patient concerns, follow-up if a delayed antibiotic prescribing plan was implemented, assess barriers to receiving their prescription, medication compliance, and identify adverse effects or possibly drug-drug interactions that were not identified in the ED.[19] Using follow-up communication as an AS tool requires investigation into current follow-up practices and collaboration with care coordinators, nurses, quality improvement representatives, or pharmacists.

De-escalation of therapy once microbiologic culture finalizes 48 hours to 72 hours after initiation of empiric antimicrobial therapy is routine in the inpatient setting but presents challenges for treating and releasing patients. Similarly, implementing initiatives surrounding the shorter is better campaign, debunking the perceived need to treat beyond resolution of symptoms to prevent relapses or prevent antibiotic resistance, has similar challenges compared with the inpatient setting.[83,84] Recent literature comparing short and long antibiotic courses for a variety of infectious diseases treated in the ED have shown similar efficacy and should be used to influence more appropriate empiric antibiotic regimens.[85] Incorporation of de-escalation activities and recommending cessation of antibiotics once symptoms have resolved, however, are not routinely incorporated into current ED ASPs. Culture surveillance and follow-up or prescription review programs could be an ideal area to integrate these initiatives to improve optimal prescribing and reduce overall unnecessary antibiotic exposure. Concerns that deescalating broad coverage or stopping antibiotic therapy may result in future inappropriate use or partial antibiotic regimens readily available to patients would need to be addressed and collaborative efforts with patients, community clinicians, and outpatient pharmacy for disposal of unused antibiotics would be necessary.

Antibiotic overuse is prevalent in pediatric emergency care in nonpediatric hospital EDs compared with freestanding children's hospital EDs.[13] Identifying key stakeholders in pediatric, general, and community EDs to engage front-line providers, pediatric disease state education, and focused guideline development and integration of these clinical pathways into the EMR are suggested strategies to target pediatric antibiotic overuse.[86] Urgent care settings are a site targeted by the CDC Core Elements of Outpatient Antibiotic Stewardship but deserve further mention.[4] An evaluation of health care claims found that 39% of 2.7 million urgent care center visits resulted in antibiotic prescribing[87]; 16% of all visits were for antibiotic-inappropriate respiratory diagnoses and almost half received antibiotics (46%). Collaboration with organization IT colleagues and health insurance companies may provide useful data on antibiotic prescribing behaviors and clinician performance to help target high-priority conditions. Two novel studies discussing remote pharmacist–led culture follow-up services to urgent care sites are described previously and highlight the need to develop AS strategies focused on decision to treat and appropriate antibiotic selection, dose, and duration in this setting.[39,40] Similarly, health care systems should consider ED ASP expansion to stand-alone or off-campus EDs and smaller community hospitals. Telemedicine and telehealth, remote EM pharmacist consultation, and state and local public health collaboratives may be novel approaches to expanding acute-care AS initiatives and improving coordination of care within and across health care systems.[4,88]

SUMMARY

The ED is a unique area of practice with several barriers but also many opportunities for AS. Strategies focused on appropriate antimicrobial use; drug selection, dose, and duration; prompt administration; and reducing ED returns and readmissions involves collaboration with a wide range of both community and acute-care colleagues to be successful. These AS interventions alone or in combination can have significant positive effects on ED patient outcomes.[89]

DISCLOSURE

Dr N.M. Acquisto has nothing to disclose. Dr L. May has the following disclosures: she has previously received research support from Cepheid and BioFire Diagnostics; she currently receives research support from Roche Diagnostics; she is an advisor to Bio-Rad, Qvella, Nabriva, and Roche Diagnostics; and she has received honoraria for speaking engagements from Cepheid.

REFERENCES

1. Fishman N. Policy statement on antimicrobial stewardship by the Society for Healthcare Epidemiology of America (SHEA), the Infectious Diseases Society of America (IDSA), and the Pediatric Infectious Diseases Society (PIDS). Infect Control Hosp Epidemiol 2012;33:322–7.
2. Barlam TF, Cosgrove SE, Abbo LM, et al. Implementing an antibiotic stewardship program: guidelines by the Infectious Diseases Society of American and the Society for Healthcare Epidemiology of America. Clin Infect Dis 2016;62:e51–77.

3. National hospital ambulatory medical care survey: 2016 Emergency department summary tables. 2016. Available at: https://www.cdc.gov/nchs/data/nhamcs/web_tables/2016_ed_web_tables.pdf. Accessed August 10, 2019.
4. Sanchez GV, Fleming-Dutra KE, Roberts RM, et al. Core elements of outpatient antibiotic stewardship. MMWR Recomm Rep 2016;65(No. RR-6):1–12.
5. Centers for Disease Control and Prevention. Office-related antibiotic prescribing for persons aged < 14 years – United States, 1993-1994 to 2007-2008. MMWR Morb Mortal Wkly Rep 2011;60:1153–85.
6. Shapiro DJ, Hicks LA, Pavia AT, et al. Antibiotic prescribing for adults in ambulatory care in the USA, 2007-09. J Antimicrob Chemother 2014;69:234–40.
7. Donnelly JP, Baddley JW, Wang HE. Antibiotic utilization for respiratory tract infections in U.S. emergency departments. Antimicrob Agents Chemother 2014; 58:1451–7.
8. Lee GC, Reveles KR, Attridge RT, et al. Outpatient antibiotic prescribing in the United States: 2000 to 2010. BMC Med 2014;12:96.
9. Fleming-Dutra KE, Hersh AL, Shapiro DJ, et al. Prevalence of inappropriate antibiotic prescriptions among US ambulatory care visits, 2010-2011. JAMA 2016;15: 1864–73.
10. Gonzales R, Camargo CA, MacKenzie T, et al. Antibiotic treatment of acute respiratory infections in acute care settings. Acad Emerg Med 2006;13:288–94.
11. Timbrook TT, Caffrey AR, Ovalle A, et al. Assessments of opportunities to improve antibiotic prescribing in an emergency department. Infect Dis Ther 2017;6: 497–505.
12. Kroening-Roche JC, Soroudi A, Catillo EM, et al. Antibiotic and bronchodilator prescribing for acute bronchitis in the emergency department. J Emerg Med 2012;43:221–7.
13. Poole NM, Shapiro DJ, Fleming-Dutra KE, et al. Antibiotic prescribing for children in United States Emergency Departments: 2009-2014. Pediatrics 2019;143: e20181056.
14. Shehab N, Lovegrove MC, Geller AI, et al. US emergency department visits for outpatient adverse drug events, 2013-2014. JAMA 2016;316:2115–25.
15. Stearns CR, Gonzales R, Camargo CA Jr, et al. Antibiotic prescriptions are associated with increased patient satisfaction with emergency visits for acute respiratory infections. Acad Emerg Med 2009;16:934–41.
16. Ong S, Nakase J, Moran GJ, et al. Antibiotic use for emergency department patients with upper respiratory infections: prescribing practices, patient expectations, and patient satisfaction. Ann Emerg Med 2007;50:213–2020.
17. Ong S, Moran GJ, Krishnadasan A, et al. Antibiotic prescribing practices of emergency physicians and patient expectations for uncomplicated lacerations. West J Emerg Med 2011;12:375–80.
18. Studdert DM, Mello MM, Sage WM, et al. Defensive medicine among high-risk specialist physicians in a volatile malpractice environment. JAMA 2005;293: 2609–17.
19. May L, Cosgrove S, L'Archeveque M, et al. A call to action for antimicrobial stewardship in the emergency department: approaches and strategies. Ann Emerg Med 2013;62:69–77.
20. Bishop BM. Antimicrobial stewardship in the emergency department: challenges, opportunities, and a call to action for pharmacists. J Pharm Pract 2016;29: 556–63.
21. Pulia M, Redwood R, May L. Antimicrobial stewardship in the emergency department. Emerg Med Clin North Am 2018;36:853–72.

22. Trinh TD, Klinger KP. Antimicrobial stewardship in the emergency department. Infect Dis Ther 2015;4:S39–50.
23. May L, Yadav K, Gaona SD, et al. MITIGATE antimicrobial stewardship toolkit. 2018. Available at: http://www.shea-online.org/images/priority-topics/MITIGATE_TOOLKIT_final.pdf. Accessed August 10, 2019.
24. Blanchette L, Gauthier T, Heil E, et al. The essential role of pharmacists in antibiotic stewardship in outpatient care: an official position statement of the Society of Infectious Diseases Pharmacists. J Am Pharm Assoc (2003) 2018;58:481–4.
25. Morgan SR, Acquisto NM, Coralic Z, et al. Clinical pharmacy services in the emergency department. Am J Emerg Med 2018;36:1727–32.
26. DeWitt KM, Weiss SJ, Rankin S, et al. Impact of an emergency medicine pharmacist on antibiotic dosing adjustment. Am J Emerg Med 2016;24:980–4.
27. Jorgensen SCJ, Yeung SL, Zurayk M, et al. Leveraging antimicrobial stewardship in the emergency department to improve the quality of urinary tract infection management and outcomes. Open Forum Infect Dis 2018;5:ofy101.
28. Attwood R. Impact of emergency department clinical pharmacist response to an automated electronic notification system on timing and appropriateness of antimicrobials in severe or septic shock in the emergency department: 332. Ann Emerg Med 2012;60:S118.
29. Moussavi K, Nikitenko V. Pharmacist impact on the time to antibiotic administration in patients with sepsis in an ED. Am J Emerg Med 2016;34:2117–21.
30. DeFrates SR, Weant KA, Seamon JP, et al. Emergency pharmacist impact on health care-associated pneumonia empiric therapy. J Pharm Pract 2013;26:125–30.
31. Kulwicki BD, Brandt KL, Wolf LM, et al. Impact of an emergency medicine pharmacist on empiric antibiotic prescribing for pneumonia and intra-abdominal infections. Am J Emerg Med 2019;37:839–44.
32. Harvey S, Hall AB, Wilson K. Impact of an emergency medicine pharmacist on initial antibiotic prophylaxis for open fractures in trauma patients. Am J Emerg Med 2018;36:290–3.
33. Acquisto NM, Baker NM. Antimicrobial stewardship in the emergency department. J Pharm Pract 2011;24:196–202.
34. Baker SN, Acquisto NM, Ashley ED, et al. Pharmacist-managed antimicrobial stewardship program for patients discharged from the emergency department. J Pharm Pract 2012;25:190–4.
35. Davis LC, Covey B, Weston JS, et al. Pharmacist-driven antimicrobial optimization in the emergency department. Am J Health Syst Pharm 2016;73:S49–56.
36. Miller K, McGraw MA, Tomsey A, et al. Pharmacist addition to post-ED review of discharge antimicrobial regimens. Am J Emerg Med 2014;32:1270–4.
37. Randolph TC, Parker A, Meyer L, et al. Effect of a pharmacist-managed culture review process on antimicrobial therapy in an emergency department. Am J Health Syst Pharm 2011;68:916–9.
38. Dumkov LE, Kenney RM, MacDonald NC, et al. Impact of a multidisciplinary culture follow-up program of antimicrobial therapy in the emergency department. Infect Dis Ther 2014;3:45–53.
39. Dumkow LE, Beuschel TS, Brandt BL. Expanding antimicrobial stewardship to urgent care centers through a pharmacist-led culture follow-up program. Infect Dis Ther 2017;6:453–9.
40. Fay LN, Wolf LM, Brandt KL, et al. Pharmacist-led antimicrobial stewardship program in an urgent care setting. Am J Health Syst Pharm 2019;76:175–81.

41. Patanwala AE, Sanders AB, Thomas MC, et al. A prospective, multicenter study of pharmacist activities resulting in medication error interception in the emergency department. Ann Emerg Med 2012;59:369–73.

42. Redefining the antibiotic stewardship team: recommendations from the American Nurses Association/Centers of Disease Control and Prevention workgroup on the role of registered nurses in hospital antibiotic stewardship practices. 2017. Available at: https://www.cdc.gov/antibiotic-use/healthcare/pdfs/ANA-CDC-whitepaper.pdf. Accessed September 1, 2019.

43. Draper HM, Farland JB, Heidel RE, et al. Comparison of bacteria isolated from emergency department patients versus hospitalized patients. Am J Health Syst Pharm 2013;70:2124–8.

44. Schempp J, Pfaff C, Lennellett E, et al. Comparison of inpatient and emergency department (ED) antibiograms in a community hospital. Crit Care Med 2017; 46:663.

45. Jorgensen S, Zurayk M, Yeung S, et al. Emergency department urinary antibiograms differ by specific patient group. J Clin Microbiol 2017;55:2629–36.

46. Nicolle LE, Gupta K, Bradley SF, et al. Clinical practice guideline for the management of asymptomatic bacteriuria: 2019 update by the Infectious Diseases Society of America. Clin Infect Dis 2019;68:e83–110.

47. Rattinger GB, Mullins CD, Zuckerman IH, et al. A sustainable strategy to prevent misuse of antibiotics for acute respiratory infections. PLoS One 2012;7:e51147.

48. Meeker D, Linder JA, Fox CR, et al. Effect of behavioral interventions on inappropriate antibiotic prescribing among primary care practices: a randomized clinical trial. JAMA 2016;315:562–70.

49. Lin G, Knowlson S, Nguyen H, et al. Urine test stewardship for catheterized patients in the critical care setting: provider perceptions and impact of electronic order set interventions. Am J Infect Control 2019. https://doi.org/10.1016/j.ajic.2019.04.005.

50. Hecker MT, Fox CJ, Son AH, et al. Effect of a stewardship intervention on adherence to uncomplicated cystitis and pyelonephritis guidelines in an emergency department setting. PLoS One 2014;9:e87899.

51. Yadav K, Meeker D, Mistry D, et al. A multifaceted intervention improves prescribing for acute respiratory infection for adults and children in emergency department and urgent care settings. Acad Emerg Med 2019;26:719–31.

52. Ayanruoh S, Waseem M, Quee F, et al. Impact of rapid streptococcal test on antibiotic use in a pediatric emergency department. Pediatr Emerg Care 2009;25: 748–50.

53. Blaschke AJ, Shapiro DJ, Pavia AT, et al. A national study of the impact of rapid influenza testing on clinical care in the emergency department. J Pediatric Infect Dis Soc 2014;3:112–8.

54. Green DA, Hitoaliaj L, Kotansky B, et al. Clinical utility of on-demand multiplex respiratory pathogen testing among adult outpatients. J Clin Microbiol 2016;54: 2950–5.

55. Schechter-Perkins EM, Mitchell PM, Nelson KP, et al. Point-of-care influenza testing does not significantly shorten time to disposition among patients with an influenza-like illness. Am J Emerg Med 2019;37:873–8.

56. Wabe N, Li L, Lindeman R, et al. The impact of rapid molecular diagnostic testing for respiratory viruses on outcomes for emergency department patients. Med J Aust 2010;210:316–20.

57. Kamath RS, Sudhakar D, Gardner JG, et al. Guidelines vs actual management of skin and soft tissue infection in the emergency department. Open Forum Infect Dis 2018;5:ofx188.

58. Acquisto NM, Bodkin RP, Brown JE, et al. MRSA nares swab is a more accurate predictor of MRSA wound infection compared with clinical risk factors in emergency department patients with skin and soft tissue infections. Emerg Med J 2018;35:357–60.

59. May LS, Rothman RE, Miller LG, et al. A randomized clinical trial comparing use of rapid molecular testing for Staphylococcus aureus for patients with cutaneous abscesses in the emergency department with standard of care. Infect Control Hosp Epidemiol 2015;36:1423–30.

60. Rivard KR, Dumkov LE, Draper HM, et al. Impact of rapid diagnostic testing for chlamydia and gonorrhea on appropriate antimicrobial utilization in the emergency department. Diagn Microbiol Infect Dis 2017;87:175–9.

61. May L, Ware CE, Jordan JA, et al. A randomized controlled trial comparing the treatment of patients tested for chlamydia and gonorrhea after a rapid polymerase chain reaction test versus standard of care testing. Sex Transm Dis 2016; 43:290–5.

62. CMS.gov. Centers for Medicare and Medicaid Services. Clinical laboratory improvement amendments (CLIA). 2019. Available at: https://www.cms.gov/Regulations-and-Guidance/Legislation/CLIA/index.html. Accessed September 4, 2019.

63. Schuetz P, Christ-Crain M, Thomann R, et al. Effect of procalcitonin-based guidelines vs. standard guidelines on antibiotic use in lower respiratory tract infections. The ProHOSP randomized controlled trial. JAMA 2009;302:1059–66.

64. Huang DT, Yealy DM, Filbin MR, et al. Procalcitonin-guided use of antibiotics for lower respiratory tract infection. N Engl J Med 2018;379:236–49.

65. Conners GP, Hays DP. Emergency department drug orders: does drug storage location make a difference? Ann Emerg Med 2007;50:414–8.

66. Murray KA, Belanger A, Devine LT, et al. Emergency department discharge prescription errors in an academic medical center. Proc (Bayl Univ Med Cent) 2017; 30:143–6.

67. Cesarz JL, Steffenhagen AL, Svenson J, et al. Emergency department discharge prescription interventions by emergency medicine pharmacists. Ann Emerg Med 2013;61:209–14.

68. Levy MM, Evans LE, Rhodes A. The surviving sepsis campaign bundle: 2018 update. Crit Care Med 2018;46:997–1000.

69. Hoff WS, Bonadies JA, Cachecho R, et al. East practice management guidelines work group: update to practice management guidelines for prophylactic antibiotic use in open fractures. J Trauma 2011;40:751–4.

70. Lack WD, Karunakar MA, Angerame MR, et al. Type III open tibia fractures: immediate antibiotic prophylaxis minimizes infection. J Orthop Trauma 2015;29:1–6.

71. Taplitz RA, Kennedy EB, Bow EJ, et al. Outpatient management of fever and neutropenia in adults treated for malignancy: American Society of Clinical Oncology and Infectious Diseases Society of American clinical practice guideline update. J Clin Oncol 2018;36:1443–53.

72. Spencer S, Ipema H, Hartke P, et al. Intravenous push administration of antibiotics: literature and considerations. Hosp Pharm 2018;53:157–69.

73. Hayes B, Zaharna L, Winters ME, et al. To-go medications for decreasing ED return visits. Am J Emerg Med 2012;30:2011–4.

74. Sarangarm D, Sarangarm P, Fleegler M, et al. Patients given take home medications instead of paper prescriptions are more likely to return to emergency department. Hosp Pharm 2017;52:438–43.
75. Mandell LA, Wunderink RG, Anzueto A, et al. Infectious Diseases Society of America/American Thoracic Society consensus guidelines on the management of community-acquired pneumonia in adults. Clin Infect Dis 2007;44:S27–72.
76. Self WH, Speroff T, Grijalva C, et al. Reducing blood culture contamination in the emergency department: an interrupted time series quality improvement study. Acad Emerg Med 2013;20:89–97.
77. Skalkos K. Blood culture contamination rates decrease using new product and practice changes. Am J Infect Control 2014;42(6):S130.
78. Rupp ME, Cavalieri J, Marolf C, et al. Reduction in blood culture contamination through use of initial specimen diversion device. Clin Infect Dis 2017;65:201–5.
79. Gander RM, Byrd L, DeCrescenzo M, et al. Impact of blood cultures drawn by phlebotomy on contamination rates and health care costs in a hospital emergency department. J Clin Microbiol 2009;47:1021–4.
80. Richter SS, Beekmann SE, Croco JL, et al. Minimizing the workup of blood culture contaminants: implementation and evaluation of a laboratory-based algorithm. J Clin Microbiol 2002;40:2437–44.
81. Kim JS, Kang GE, Kim HS, et al. Evaluation of verigene blood culture test systems for rapid identification of positive blood cultures. Biomed Res Int 2016;2016: 1081536.
82. Lagacé-Wiens PRS, Adams HJ, Karlowsky JA, et al. Identification of blood culture isolates directly from positive blood cultures by use of matrix-assisted laser desorption ionization-time of flight mass spectrometry and a commercial extraction system: analysis of performance, cost, and turnaround time. J Clin Microbiol 2012;50:3324–8.
83. Spellberg B. The new antibiotic mantra-"shorter is better". JAMA Intern Med 2016;176:1254–5.
84. Spellberg B. The maturing antibiotic mantra: "shorter is still better". J Hosp Med 2018;13:361–2.
85. Spellberg B, Rice LB. Duration of antibiotic therapy: shorter is better. Ann Intern Med 2019;171:210–1.
86. Mistry RD, May LS, Pulia MS. Improving antimicrobial stewardship in pediatric emergency care: a pathway forward. Pediatrics 2019;143:e20182972.
87. Palms DL, Hicks LA, Bartoces M. Comparison of antibiotic prescribing in retail clinics, urgent care centers, emergency departments, and traditional ambulatory care settings in the United States. JAMA Intern Med 2018;178:1267–9.
88. California Department of Public Health. Emergency department antibiotic stewardship collaborative. 2018. Available at: https://www.cdph.ca.gov/Programs/CHCQ/HAI/Pages/EmergencyDeptCollaborative.aspx. Accessed August 15, 2019.
89. Losier M, Ramsey TD, Wilby KJ, et al. A systematic review of antimicrobial stewardship interventions in the emergency department. Ann Pharmacother 2017;51: 774–90.

Recommendations for Improving Antimicrobial Stewardship in Long-Term Care Settings Through Collaboration

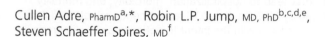

Cullen Adre, PharmD[a],*, Robin L.P. Jump, MD, PhD[b,c,d,e],
Steven Schaeffer Spires, MD[f]

KEYWORDS

- Antimicrobial stewardship • Long-term care facilities • Collaboration
- Antibiotic resistance • *Clostridioides difficile*

KEY POINTS

- Long-term care settings face many barriers to implementing effective antimicrobial stewardship programs.
- Collaboration with regional acute care hospital patient share networks, public health departments, and laboratories can offset these barriers.
- Effective partnerships with pharmacists, prescribers, and nurses in these settings can reduce the variability in education and improve the effectiveness of antimicrobial stewardship interventions.

INTRODUCTION

Postacute and long-term care (LTC) settings are an increasingly important part of health care systems. In the United States, some 15,700 LTC settings care for more than 4 million people annually.[1] As the general population ages, the use of LTC will continue to increase, with some estimates projecting that nearly half of people aged 65 years and older will spend time in a nursing home.[2] According to the Centers for

[a] Tennessee Department of Health, Andrew Johnson Tower, 3.417C, 710 James Robertson Parkway, Nashville, TN 37243, USA; [b] Geriatric Research Education and Clinical Center (GRECC); [c] Specialty Care Center of Innovation at the VA Northeast Ohio Healthcare System, Cleveland, OH, USA; [d] Division of Infectious Diseases and HIV Medicine, Department of Medicine, Case Western Reserve University School of Medicine, 10900 Euclid Avenue, Cleveland, OH 44106, USA; [e] Department of Population and Quantitative Health Sciences, Case Western Reserve University School of Medicine, 10900 Euclid Avenue, Cleveland, OH 44106, USA; [f] Duke Center for Antimicrobial Stewardship and Infection Prevention, Division of Infectious Diseases, Duke University School of Medicine, DUMC PO Box 102359, Durham, NC 27710, USA
* Corresponding author.
E-mail address: Cullen.adre@tn.gov

Infect Dis Clin N Am 34 (2020) 129–143
https://doi.org/10.1016/j.idc.2019.10.007
0891-5520/20/Published by Elsevier Inc.

id.theclinics.com

Disease Control and Prevention (CDC), up to 70% of residents in LTC facilities (LTCFs) receive an antibiotic each year.[3] A significant proportion of these are unnecessary and up to 75% are prescribed inappropriately.[4,5] Unnecessary prescribing (eg, for asymptomatic bacteriuria) not only increases the potential for patient harms, such as adverse drug events and *Clostridioides* (formerly *Clostridium*) *difficile* infections (CDIs) but also contributes to the prevalence of multidrug-resistant organisms (MDROs). The consequences of acquiring an MDRO range from colonization, necessitating contact precautions in order to reduce the risk of transmission to other residents, to infections that are difficult to treat and may lead to hospitalization, morbidity, and mortality.

To mitigate the threats posed by MDROs, the CDC recommends adoption of 7 core elements for antimicrobial stewardship with the intent to optimize antibiotic prescribing and to decrease morbidity associated with poor prescribing practices.[6] Furthermore, the Centers for Medicare and Medicaid Services (CMS) recently revised the conditions of participation, requiring LTC facilities to have an antimicrobial stewardship program that includes antibiotic use protocols and a system for monitoring antibiotic use.[7] However, LTC faces many challenges and barriers to implementing antimicrobial stewardship programs, including:

- Constrained financial resources
- Insufficient training in antimicrobial stewardship principles and practices
- Limited access to infectious disease–trained physicians and pharmacists
- Little capacity for on-site diagnostic test and laboratory studies
- High rates of staff turnover, which hinder efforts for education and contribute to deficits in the overall institutional memory

When viewing LTCs as part of the continuum of health care, these same challenges and barriers become opportunities for collaborative efforts to build successful antimicrobial stewardship programs. Collaboration can, and should, occur at the level of health care facilities and systems, with public health departments, with laboratory partners, and among personnel including nursing staff, prescribers, and pharmacists. This article discusses the potential for collaborative efforts to improve the success of LTC settings as they incorporate antimicrobial stewardship into their settings while continuing to deliver safe, high-quality care for their residents.

COLLABORATION AMONG HEALTH CARE FACILITIES AND SYSTEMS

If lack of resources is the "poison" that prevents effective antimicrobial stewardship, then collaboration is the antidote. LTC settings and acute care hospitals (ACHs) are already enmeshed through shared patients. LTC settings rely heavily on regional ACHs for their referrals, and any system-level efforts to strengthen that connectivity are typically welcomed. In general, most ACHs have successfully implemented antimicrobial stewardship programs that meet the 7 core elements and 95% of them have engaged in at least 1 action to improve antimicrobial use.[8] Furthermore, ACHs are already held accountable for health care–associated infections such as CDI and methicillin-resistant *Staphylococcus aureus* bloodstream infections. The likelihood of developing these infections, or those caused by other MDROs, depends in part on the prevalence of those organisms in the community, including in LTC settings.[9,10] Thus, it behooves both LTC settings and ACHs to collaborate with their regional partners.

Health care–associated CDI shows the interconnectedness of acute and LTC settings. Brown and colleagues[11] conducted a retrospective multilevel cohort study to examine the drivers of CDI in 130 ACHs and 121 LTC settings in the Veterans Affairs

(VA) health care system. Recent ACH exposure was a strong risk factor for developing CDI (unadjusted incidence risk ratio of 4.84; 95% confidence interval, 4.34–5.31). Thus, the ACHs were strong contributors to the subsequent risk of CDI in LTC settings, with some patients afflicted with CDI in LTC requiring hospitalization. Similarly, Simmering and colleagues[12] found that the rate of CDI among LTC residents increased with both the number of patients transferred from ACHs and the number of different ACHs sending patients to LTC. The outcomes from this study emphasize that regional networks and their interconnectedness influence the rates of CDI, with the subsequent implication that addressing antimicrobial stewardship programs and infection prevention and control efforts across these networks have the potential to reduce regional CDI rates.

Outcomes from an intervention to reduce increasing rates of CDI at a 185-bed county hospital provide a real-world perspective on collaboration between LTC settings and their affiliated county hospital (Steven Schaeffer Spires, unpublished data, 2018). An abrupt increase in CDI cases prompted development of a robust CDI prevention taskforce within a county hospital. In the next quarter, the number of hospital-onset CDI cases decreased by nearly 50%, returning to the previous baseline of less than 4 cases per 10,000 patient days (**Fig. 1**). Recognizing that these hospital-onset CDI cases were influenced by events occurring in postacute and LTC settings, a team from the county hospital developed a regional collaboration with the 6 main LTC facilities associated with the county hospital. The antimicrobial stewardship team from the county hospital (ASTCH) began by appealing to the LTC settings' desire for connectivity, offering free and contracted services to address both their antimicrobial usage and certain infection prevention strategies. Services included in-person so-called chalk talks, free education accredited at the county hospital, assistance with diagnostic stewardship, and providing an antibiogram. The ASTCH also created "report cards" for each provider that summarized the antibiotics they prescribed to patients with asymptomatic bacteriuria as well as the number of patients who received antibiotics for any indication and went on to develop CDI in the following 28 days. For providers who were clear outliers regarding their treatment of asymptomatic bacteriuria, the ASTCH also offered peer-to-peer "cup of coffee" interventions.[13] Both the number of antibiotics prescribed for asymptomatic bacteriuria and the total number of antimicrobial starts by LTC providers decreased; these changes were sustained for

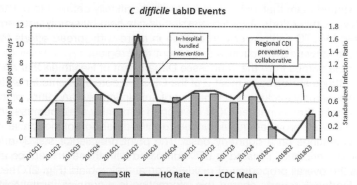

Fig. 1. Changes in the rate of CDI laboratory identified (LabID) events. Following initiation of a bundled intervention at a county hospital, the rate of hospital-onset (HO) *C difficile* LabID events per 10,000 patient days (*red line*) and the standard infection ratio (SIR) (*brown bars*) decreased. Later, implementation of a regional CDI prevention collaborative saw further decreases, below that of the previous baseline.

12 months following completion of the intervention. Collaboration between 6 LTC settings and the county hospital led to a measurable and sustained reduction in CDI throughout the region, providing a strong example of successful collaboration to improve health care outcomes.

Similar to *C difficile*, carbapenem-resistant Enterobacteriaceae (CRE) have also been spread among acute and LTC settings by shared patients. Won and colleagues[14] described the regional spread of *Klebsiella pneumoniae* carbapenemase-producing organisms (KPCs) in the Chicago, Illinois, metropolitan region. Their investigation revealed that 60% of KPC cases were related to a single long-term acute care hospital, which likely related to the convergence of several medically complex patients who required long-term stays in a setting that could provide ventilatory support. An additional 26% of cases seemed to result from exposure to other LTC settings; only 10% of cases were related to ACH exposure. In response to these CRE outbreaks, the Illinois Department of Public Health created an extensively drug-resistant organism (XDRO) registry (www.xdro.org) and, in 2013, made CRE reportable.[15] This registry receives weekly automated reports from more than 170 facilities across the state and allows MDRO information to be shared with individual facilities. Through social network analysis, Ray and colleagues[16] were able to predict CRE rates for these individual facilities within this network in Illinois. By measuring a facility's risk for admitting patients with CRE and the potential for transfer of those individuals within a network, targeted interventions can be developed to mitigate the regional spread of MDROs.

COLLABORATION WITH PUBLIC HEALTH

Previous work has described the clear need for effective antimicrobial stewardship in LTC.[6,17–20] However, specific guidance for effective implementation of antimicrobial stewardship programs in LTC settings is not yet well established.[19,21] Collaboration can help LTC settings create successful and sustainable antimicrobial stewardship programs, particularly with partners that are knowledgeable and sympathetic to LTC. Departments of health are perfectly positioned to provide guidance, resources, and support (all free of charge) to help LTC settings provide health care while also serving as homes to their residents. However, interactions with surveyors have led to the perception of public health offices only as regulatory bodies, overlooking the breadth and depth of resources available. Many health departments have a health care–associated team that includes individuals specifically detailed to bolster antimicrobial stewardship efforts. These professionals can help by simply answering questions posed by LTC settings or can engage in more widespread efforts to support antimicrobial stewardship activities throughout their region.

An example comes from the Tennessee Department of Health (DOH), which found that LTC settings struggled to meet 2 of the CDC's 7 core elements for antimicrobial stewardship, namely tracking and reporting of antibiotic use (C.A., unpublished data). To address this, the Tennessee DOH developed a monthly antibiotic use point prevalence survey and provided individualized reports detailing antibiotic use in participating LTC settings on a quarterly basis. The point prevalence survey queried the proportion of antibiotics initiated in LTC compared with those present on admission as well as the overall proportion of residents on antimicrobials (**Fig. 2**). The resulting quarterly feedback reports shared this information in a concise format that allowed each LTC setting to compare its antibiotic use with the average use throughout Tennessee. In addition to helping participating LTC settings meet the core elements, the quarterly reports from the Tennessee DOH helped guide local antimicrobial stewardship efforts.

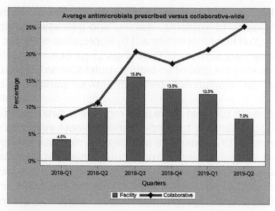

Fig. 2. Excerpt from a Tennessee Department of Health Antibiotic Use Point Prevalence Survey Sample Report. The blue bars represent the average percentage of a facility's patients who were on antimicrobials for specific quarters (Q). This percentage is contrasted with a red line, which is the average percentage of all reporting facilities' patients who were on antimicrobials for specific quarters. This contrast allows facilities to see and trend how their antibiotic use compares with that of their peers.

Public health departments can provide incentives and encouragement for facilities that are meeting conditions of participation. The Minnesota Department of Health created an antimicrobial stewardship honor roll specifically for LTC settings (**Table 1**).[22] The benefits from this antimicrobial stewardship honor roll include a

Table 1
Minnesota long-term care honor roll requirements table

Status Level	Requirements

Bronze (commitment)	• Facility antibiotic stewardship policy
	• Description of antibiotic use protocols
	• Description of a system to track antibiotic use
	• Letter from an administrative leader
	• Statement of commitment and policy
	• Names of stewardship leaders and positions of team members
	• Description of (at minimum) yearly education for prescribers that includes:
	  ○ Dates of recent/upcoming training
	  ○ Targeted staff
	  ○ Attendance rate

Silver (action)	• Achievement of bronze-level requirements for commitment • At least 1 action for resident/family/public education about antibiotic use • At least 1 additional intervention action implemented to improve antibiotic use
Gold (collaboration)	• Achievement of bronze-level and silver-level requirements for commitment and action • Looking beyond their facility to practice stewardship in a formal collaborative way

Courtesy of Long-term Care Honor Roll: One Health Antibiotic Stewardship Collaborative, Minnesota Department of Health, St. Paul, MN; with permission.

tangible certification or seal of approval from the department of health, which LTC settings can proudly display to residents, visitors, and their staff members; this kind of positive recognition can bolster commitment to appropriate antibiotic use. In addition, the honor roll program encourages LTC settings to go beyond meeting the basic requirements (ie, checking the box) of an antimicrobial stewardship program and strive instead to foster an institutional commitment to patient safety and quality improvement.

Departments of health can also serve as a region's bulletin board, using their relationships with multiple partners to support and promote initiatives and events. For example, the Tennessee DOH created a monthly antimicrobial stewardship and infection control call; all interested parties from acute, long-term, and outpatient settings are invited to participate. Cycling every month between topics specific to antimicrobial stewardship and infection prevention and control, the call offers an open forum to encourage discussion and highlight successful efforts by participating settings (**Table 2**). Additional benefits from the call include updating participants about regulatory changes, making recommendations on how to adhere to those changes, and sharing success stories from LTC settings that have found ways to overcome common barriers. In addition, the Tennessee DOH uses the monthly calls to compile an updated LISTSERV for antimicrobial stewardship champions at the participating LTC settings; the LISTSERV functions as a network and resource for its diverse members, which include infection preventionists, directors of nursing, pharmacists, medical directors, and infectious disease physicians.

COLLABORATION AMONG NURSES AND PRESCRIBERS

Nurses are instrumental to successful antimicrobial stewardship programs in any setting and especially in LTC. A joint publication from the American Nurses Association and CDC reviewed antimicrobial stewardship programs and the current state of antibiotic resistance.[23] The publication details opportunities for nurses to add their expertise to antimicrobial stewardship efforts and makes several strong recommendations to incorporate these principles into nursing education. In LTC settings, nurses and nurse assistants are the central point of contact between clinicians, allied health service providers, administration, ancillary staff, residents, and their family members. Especially when supported with education and experience, nurses and nurse

Table 2 Topics addressed in monthly calls offered by the Tennessee Department of Health	
Antimicrobial Stewardship	**Infection Prevention and Control**
Polypharmacy and its effect on antimicrobial usage in the elderly population	NHSN enrollment process
Asymptomatic bacteriuria protocols	NHSN process measures modules
Disease of the month[a]	Infection prevention and the role of the environment
Respiratory infections	Nursing home prevalence survey updates
Core element intervention reviews	Infection control tag reviews by a state surveyor
NHSN urinary tract infection protocol	NHSN LTC facility dashboard Interfacility transfer communication

Abbreviation: NHSN, National Health and Safety Network.
[a] Some topics addressed both antimicrobial stewardship and infection control and prevention.

assistants are well positioned to serve as powerful advocates to incorporate antimicrobial stewardship into daily practice.

High rates of staff turnover coupled with limited time and resources in LTC are both cogent barriers to nurses' involvement in antimicrobial stewardship efforts. An unfortunate consequence of the frequent influx of nurses and nurse assistants new to individual LTC settings is that more involved or complicated topics, such as antimicrobial stewardship, occasionally concede to fundamental topics like hand hygiene and falls prevention. However, for nurses in LTC settings, education increases their confidence to engage in antimicrobial stewardship practices.[24] For example, if the team decides to take an active monitoring approach, nurses can help educate the resident and family about the rationale for avoiding a potentially unnecessary medication while offering supportive care. For nurses who are not comfortable with these conversations, coaching and role playing may help them gain confidence. As nursing practice evolves to meet the changing health care landscape, nurses must be equipped with the necessary additional knowledge and expertise.

Prescribers working in LTC settings tend to have a wide variability in how they use antimicrobials, and resident characteristics account for few of those differences.[11,25,26] As for nurses, prescribers also need regular education tailored to their training that addresses the following:

- Potential risks and benefits of antibiotics
- Strengths and weaknesses of different classes of agents
- Appropriate indications and technique for collecting microbiological specimens
- Differentiation between clinical infection and colonization
- Interpretation of microbiological culture results
- The prevalence and risks associated with MDROs and C difficile

Training should be given at least annually and documented appropriately as required by CMS. In addition to formal courses, some which include certification (Table 3), a wide array of free resources are available through the CDC, the Agency for Healthcare Quality and Research (AHRQ), as well as state departments of health and some academic organizations.[21]

Furthermore, for prescribers, peer accountability is often a powerful tool for both education and practice improvement. In our experience, the first argument against most feedback reports tends to question the validity of the data comprising the metric followed by an argument for the validity of the metric itself. Appropriate risk adjustment for patients and developing a metric that is readily understood by providers is important. An example of a metric designed to improve appropriate antibiotic use might be treatment of asymptomatic bacteriuria per residents admitted. Other examples include each prescriber's days of antibiotic therapy per bed days of care or the number of antibiotic starts per month or days worked. Although these are not perfect measures, they provide a transparent, objective evaluation. Hallsworth and colleagues[27] observed a change in prescriber practices following letters sent by the Chief Medical Officer for England to clinicians prescribing antimicrobials at a rate higher than 80% of practices in the same region. In the 6-month period after 3227 letters were mailed to 784 practices, the intervention group prescribed antibiotics at a lower rate compared with the control group (126.98 per 1000 population vs 131.25 per 1000 population, or 3% relative difference), preventing an estimated 73,000 antibiotics from being dispensed. The credibility of a high-profile peer and the information about regional prescribing patterns provided a social norm that helped change prescribing behavior.

Because prescribers in LTC settings are not typically in the building on a daily basis, they must rely on communication from nurses. Effective communication requires a

Table 3	
Courses and certifications for antimicrobial stewardship	
Organization	Link
CDC	https://www.cdc.gov/antibiotic-use/community/for-hcp/continuing-education.html
AHRQ Nursing Home Antimicrobial Stewardship Guide	https://www.ahrq.gov/nhguide/index.html
APIC trainings and resources	https://apic.org/Resources/Topic-specific-infection-prevention/Antimicrobial-stewardship/
Stanford University	https://med.stanford.edu/cme/learning-opportunities/antimicrobialstewardship.html
Making a Difference Infectious Diseases Online $	http://www.mad-id.org
Society of Infectious Diseases Pharmacists $	http://bit.ly/2avkxe0
SHEA $	http://www.stewardship-education.org/education/

$ denotes cost.

Abbreviations: AHRQ, Agency for Healthcare Research and Quality; APIC, Association for Professionals in Infection Control and Epidemiology; SHEA, Society for Healthcare Epidemiology of America.

relationship grounded in mutual trust and respect; fear or lack of trust stifles effective communication to the detriment of resident care in general, not just antibiotic use. LTC settings with less hierarchical organizational structure that facilitates effective interdisciplinary communication seem to have lower rates of antimicrobial use.[19,28,29] Efforts that foster multidisciplinary communication are likely to be more effective than those targeting only prescribers or nurses alone. The authors advocate incorporating antimicrobial stewardship into other activities, such as new admissions, change of shift, wound care rounds, daily stand-ups, and prescribers' rounds. This approach can help establish the practice pattern of addressing appropriate antibiotic use on a daily basis and weaves those values into the fabric of the institutional culture.

For unplanned events, such as a change in condition or concerns raised by a family member, the authors suggest using SBAR (situation, background, assessment, and recommendation) as a standardized framework for concise communication that helps nurses talk so that prescribers will listen. SBAR provides a framework that highlights pertinent information that should be assessed and communicated when discussing a resident's change in condition. AHRQ provides a free toolkit with an SBAR form for changes in condition specifically around suspected urinary tract infection.[30] The toolkit includes training materials to help nurses gather relevant information and a structured framework for communicating that information. Using SBAR may help foster teamwork while supporting a culture centered on resident safety.

A pilot program offered through the Tennessee DOH used SBAR to help reduce asymptomatic bacteriuria in an LTC setting (C.A., unpublished data). The initiative began with education for nurses about interpreting urine culture results in the context of resident symptoms to help differentiate between colonization and infection. The next phase saw implementation of AHRQ's SBAR form for suspected urinary tract infection, which nurses filled out before calling the prescribers. This form, which uses a series of checkboxes and algorithms in the assessment section, helped guide decisions about the appropriateness of ordering a urinalysis and culture. If the predetermined criteria were not met, the nurses would engage in active monitoring of the resident and consider other reasons for a change in condition. The process of using the SBAR form streamlined and augmented communication between nurses and prescribers, letting the latter feel comfortable that they would be alerted to acute changes and helping decrease their proclivity to order an antibiotic just in case.

COLLABORATION WITH LABORATORY

The last several years have seen remarkable advancements in the diagnosis and treatment of infections. In spite of, and sometimes because of, these changes, infectious diseases diagnostics can seem like mystical phenomena, even to experienced infectious disease clinicians. Collaboration with the laboratory can help prescribers and nurses working in LTC settings improve their approach to ordering tests, collecting specimens, and interpreting results. Although rapid diagnostics and molecular assays are now integrated into the microbiology laboratory, variations in resources and expertise may influence whether and how those tests are used in any given locality.

Interpretation of microbiological results also presents challenges. For example, some clinicians may misinterpret the susceptibility results in the resident with simple cystitis caused by the *Escherichia coli* isolate shown in **Fig. 3**. Although the organism is susceptible to all of the antibiotics listed, some providers may think that ciprofloxacin is superior because it has the lowest minimum inhibitory concentration (MIC). However, MICs are not comparable between antibiotic classes, any more than 10 mg of lisinopril, furosemide, or hydrochlorothiazide would be expected to have the same influence on reducing blood pressure. Collaboration with the laboratory to remove the MICs and include only the interpretation (S for susceptible, R for resistant, and I for intermediate) may be a strong adjunct to education that stresses selection of narrow-spectrum antibiotics. Furthermore, susceptibility results from microbiological cultures should be reviewed for the opportunity to de-escalate antibiotics and an infection preventionist should be alerted to the positive cultures because recovery of MDROs may warrant contact precautions. An ideal situation would be to have laboratory results automatically integrated into LTC settings' electronic medical records; this may become reality in the future.

Most LTC settings do not have an on-site laboratory unless they are physically connected to an ACH. Accordingly, point-of-care diagnostics or next-day phlebotomy services tend to be the standard. Understanding recommendations for sample collection as well as how the laboratory processes samples may help LTC settings prioritize

>100,000 CFU/ML ESCHERICHIA COLI

	MIC	INTP	
AMPICILLIN	4	S	MCG/ML
CEFAZOLIN	<=4	S	MCG/ML
CIPROFLOXACIN	<=0.25	S	MCG/ML
TRIMETH/SULFA	<=20	S	MCG/ML
NITROFURANTOIN	<=16	S	MCG/ML
AMPICILLIN/SULB	<=2	S	MCG/ML

Fig. 3. Sample report from a urinary culture growing more than 100,000 colony-forming units (CFU) per milliliter of *E coli*. The microbiology laboratory uses the minimum inhibitory concentrations (MICs) to determine whether bacterial isolate is susceptible (S) or resistant (R) to specific antibiotics. In routine practice, clinicians should not use the MIC when choosing an antibiotic. They should choose narrow-spectrum agents to which the bacterium is susceptible.

specific tests. For microbiological samples, such as urine cultures or stool sent for *C difficile* testing, refrigeration is important both following collection as well as during transport to the laboratory. For tests typically ordered for more acute concerns, such as blood cultures or procalcitonin, the time from sample collection to results may be too long to have a meaningful influence on resident care. Furthermore, the inclination to order some tests may be a strong indicator to consider transfer to an acute care setting, provided that is consistent with the resident's goals of care.

Perhaps the most important opportunity for collaboration between an LTCF and its contracted laboratory is for the development of an antibiogram, which helps clinicians know the most common pathogens implicated for common infections and their susceptibilities to the available antibiotics.[31] LTC settings may have organisms similar to or different from other LTC and ACH settings in their region.[32,33] The Clinical and Laboratory Standards Institute calls for at least 30 isolates of an individual bacterial species in order to develop an antibiogram for that species[34]; most LTC settings cannot meet this requirement. One reasonable option to increase the number of isolates used to construct an antibiogram is to extend the collection period to 2 years. Another is to combine pathogens coming from the same source, such as all gram-negative bacteria recovered from urine cultures. This approach may be particularly appealing when a clinician is choosing an antibiotic for empiric treatment. If this level of customization is not available, then gaining access to an antibiogram from an affiliated ACH in the same region may provide some guidance.

COLLABORATION WITH PHARMACY

Drug expertise is one of the CDC's core elements of antimicrobial stewardship in LTCFs. Pharmacists have extensive drug expertise and can both lead and strengthen LTC antimicrobial stewardship programs. Most LTC settings have a consultant pharmacist, with some settings making use of remote consultation through facility networks or telepharmacy. The potential benefits to resident safety can justify the short expense of formal antimicrobial stewardship training for pharmacists. Larger LTC settings or those within networks may consider incorporating a requirement for antimicrobial stewardship certification for their pharmacists. Renegotiating contracts to include reimbursement for pharmacy services that aid in advancing antimicrobial stewardship efforts within the facility can help prompt consulting agencies to encourage certification of pharmacists.

Specific opportunities for pharmacists to support antimicrobial stewardship practices in LTC settings include development and implementation of evidence-based protocols and providing audit and feedback for prescribers. Facility-specific protocols for common infections should be grounded in evidence-based recommendations from authoritative bodies and tailored to the LTC setting's formulary, antibiogram, and practice patterns (**Table 4**). Protocols could be posted at central locations such as nurse's stations and rendered into ready-made pocket quick guides on antibiotic use that prescribers and nurses can carry with them.

Implementation of a facility-wide protocol lays the foundation for audit and feedback. As they review medications, consultant pharmacists may take the opportunity to assess whether antibiotics prescribed for specific indications were in accordance with the facility protocols. Results from these assessments can be incorporated into monthly or quarterly reviews of individual prescribers and the facility overall. Other pharmacist-led interventions that are amenable to collaboration include antibiotic timeouts, conversion from intravenous to oral antibiotics, and assisting with creating and interpreting antibiograms. Antibiotic timeouts set an expectation for nurses and

Table 4
Evidence-based resources and guidelines to aid in development of LTC antibiotic use protocols

Title	Reference
Resources that Address Several Common Infections	
Development of Minimum Criteria for the Initiation of Antibiotics in Residents of Long-term-care Facilities: Results of a Consensus Conference	Loeb et al,[36] 2001
Clinical Practice Guideline for the Evaluation of Fever and Infection in Older Adult Residents of Long-term Care Facilities: 2008 Update by the Infectious Diseases Society of America	High et al,[37] 2009
Infectious Diseases in Older Adults of Long-Term Care Facilities: Update on Approach to Diagnosis and Management	Jump et al,[38] 2018
Urinary Tract Infections and Asymptomatic Bacteriuria	
International Clinical Practice Guidelines for the Treatment of Acute Uncomplicated Cystitis and Pyelonephritis in Women: A 2010 Update by the Infectious Diseases Society of America and the European Society for Microbiology and Infectious Diseases	Gupta et al,[39] 2011
Clinical Practice Guideline for the Management of Asymptomatic Bacteriuria: 2019 Update by the Infectious Diseases Society of America	Nicolle et al,[40] 2019
Diagnosis, Prevention, and Treatment of Catheter-associated Urinary Tract Infection in Adults: 2009 International Clinical Practice Guidelines from the Infectious Diseases Society of America	Hooton et al,[41] 2010
Other Common Infections	
Clinical Practice Guidelines for *Clostridium difficile* Infection in Adults and Children: 2017 Update by the Infectious Diseases Society of America (IDSA) and Society for Healthcare Epidemiology of America (SHEA)	McDonald et al,[42] 2018
Management of Adults with Hospital-acquired and Ventilator-associated Pneumonia: 2016 Clinical Practice Guidelines by the Infectious Diseases Society of America and the American Thoracic Society	Kalil et al,[43] 2016
Infectious Diseases Society of America/American Thoracic Society Consensus Guidelines on the Management of Community-acquired Pneumonia in Adults	Mandell et al,[44] 2007
Practice Guidelines for the Diagnosis and Management of Skin and Soft-Tissue Infections	Stevens et al,[45] 2005
2012 Infectious Diseases Society of America Clinical Practice Guideline for the Diagnosis and Treatment of Diabetic Foot Infections	Lipsky et al,[46] 2012
Clinical Practice Guidelines by the Infectious Diseases Society of America for the Treatment of Methicillin-resistant *Staphylococcus aureus* Infections in Adults and Children	Liu et al,[47] 2011

prescribers to reassess the resident 2 to 3 days after an antibiotic start and to review results of microbiological cultures to determine whether antibiotics are still indicated or may be de-escalated. Pharmacists can also help work with contracted laboratories in developing a facility-specific or regional antibiograms. Consulting pharmacists can provide guidance for prescribers and nurses as they learn to interpret and use antibiograms. In a systematic review of pharmacist-involved interventions, it was found that "antimicrobial stewardship programs involving pharmacists are effective in decreasing antibiotic prescribing and increasing guideline-adherent antibiotic prescribing."[35]

SUMMARY

As LTC residents become more medically complex, collaboration becomes increasingly important. The limited resources common to most LTC settings becomes an opportunity to engage with several different partners, including regional health care networks, public health, nurses, prescribers, laboratories, and pharmacists. Collaboration to improve antimicrobial stewardship in LTC settings can enhance resident safety and lead to benefits that extend across the continuum of care.

ACKNOWLEDGMENTS AND FUNDING

This work was supported in part by funds and facilities provided by the Cleveland Geriatric Research Education and Clinical Center (GRECC) and the Specialty Care Center of Innovation at the VA Northeast Ohio Healthcare System. The findings and conclusions in this article are those of the authors, who are responsible for its content, and do not necessarily represent the views of the Department of Veterans Affairs or of the United States government.

CONFLICTS OF INTEREST

None of the authors have relevant conflicts of interest to disclose. R.L.P. Jump has received research funding from the Steris Corporation, Accelerate Diagnostics and Pfizer; she has also participated in advisory boards for Pfizer and Merck.

REFERENCES

1. Harris-Kojetin L, Sengupta M, Park-Lee E, et al. Long-term care services in the United States: 2013 overview. Vital Health Stat 3 2013;(37):1–107.
2. Spillman B, Lubitz J. New estimates of lifetime nursing home use: have patterns of use changed? Med Care 2002;40(10):965–75.
3. Nicolle LE, Bentley DW, Garibaldi R, et al. Antimicrobial use in long term–care facilities. Infect Control Hosp Epidemiol 2000;21(8):537–45.
4. Peron EP, Hirsch AA, Jury LA, et al. Another setting for stewardship: high rate of unnecessary antimicrobial use in a veterans affairs long-term care facility. J Am Geriatr Soc 2013;61(2):289–90.
5. Lim CJ, Kong DCM, Stuart RL. Reducing inappropriate antibiotic prescribing in the residential care setting: current perspectives. Clin Interv Aging 2014;9: 165–77.
6. The core elements of antibiotic stewardship for nursing homes | nursing homes and assisted living (LTC). Atlanta (GA): US Department of Health and Human Services, CDC; 2015. Available at: http://www.cdc.gov/longtermcare/index.html.
7. Medicare and Medicaid Programs. Reform of requirements for long-term care facilities. Federal Register; 2016.
8. O'Leary EN, van Santen KL, Webb AK, et al. Uptake of antibiotic stewardship programs in US acute care hospitals: findings from the 2015 National Healthcare Safety Network Annual Hospital Survey. Clin Infect Dis 2017;65(10):1748–50.

9. Dubberke ER, Reske KA, Yan Y, et al. Clostridium difficile–associated disease in a setting of endemicity: identification of novel risk factors. Clin Infect Dis 2007; 45(12):1543–9.
10. Ajao AO, Harris AD, Roghmann M-C, et al. Systematic review of measurement and adjustment for colonization pressure in studies of methicillin-resistant staphylococcus aureus, vancomycin-resistant enterococci, and clostridium difficile acquisition. Infect Control Hosp Epidemiol 2011;32(5):481–9.
11. Brown KA, Daneman N, Jones M, et al. The drivers of acute and long-term care clostridium difficile infection rates: a retrospective multilevel cohort study of 251 facilities. Clin Infect Dis 2017;65(8):1282–8.
12. Simmering JE, Tang F, Cavanaugh JE, et al. The increase in hospitalizations for urinary tract infections and the associated costs in the United States, 1998–2011. Open Forum Infect Dis 2017;4(1):ofw281.
13. Hickson GB, Pichert JW, Webb LE, et al. A complementary approach to promoting professionalism: identifying, measuring, and addressing unprofessional behaviors. Acad Med 2007;82(11):1040–8.
14. Won SY, Munoz-Price LS, Lolans K, et al. Emergence and rapid regional spread of klebsiella pneumoniae carbapenemase–producing enterobacteriaceae. Clin Infect Dis 2011;53(6):532–40.
15. Trick WE, Lin MY, Cheng-Leidig R, et al. Electronic public health registry of extensively drug-resistant organisms, Illinois, USA. Emerg Infect Dis 2015;21(10): 1725–32.
16. Ray MJ, Lin MY, Weinstein RA, et al. Spread of carbapenem-resistant enterobacteriaceae among Illinois Healthcare Facilities: the role of patient sharing. Clin Infect Dis 2016;63(7):889–93.
17. Lim CJ, Kwong M, Stuart RL, et al. Antimicrobial stewardship in residential aged care facilities: need and readiness assessment. BMC Infect Dis 2014;14(1):410.
18. Crnich CJ, Jump R, Trautner B, et al. Optimizing antibiotic stewardship in nursing homes: a narrative review and recommendations for improvement. Drugs Aging 2015;32(9):699–716.
19. Katz MJ, Gurses AP, Tamma PD, et al. Implementing antimicrobial stewardship in long-term care settings: an integrative review using a human factors approach. Clin Infect Dis 2017;65(11):1943–51.
20. McElligott M, Welham G, Pop-Vicas A, et al. Antibiotic stewardship in nursing facilities. Infect Dis Clin North Am 2017;31(4):619–38.
21. Jump RLP, Gaur S, Katz MJ, et al. Template for an antibiotic stewardship policy for post-acute and long-term care settings. J Am Med Dir Assoc 2017;18(11): 913–20.
22. Long-term Care Honor Roll: One Health Antibiotic Stewardship Collaborative. MN Department of Health.
23. Redefining the Antibiotic Stewardship Team: Recommendations from the American Nurses Association/Centers for Disease Control and Prevention Workgroup on the Role of Registered Nurses in Hospital Antibiotic Stewardship Practices. Available at: https://www.cdc.gov/antibiotic-use/healthcare/pdfs/ANA-CDC-white paper.pdf.
24. Wilson BM, Shick S, Carter RR, et al. An online course improves nurses' awareness of their role as antimicrobial stewards in nursing homes. Am J Infect Control 2017;45(5):466–70.
25. Phillips CD, Adepoju O, Stone N, et al. Asymptomatic bacteriuria, antibiotic use, and suspected urinary tract infections in four nursing homes. BMC Geriatr 2012; 12:73.

26. Daneman N, Bronskill SE, Gruneir A, et al. Variability in antibiotic use across nursing homes and the risk of antibiotic-related adverse outcomes for individual residents. JAMA Intern Med 2015;175(8):1331–9.

27. Hallsworth M, Chadborn T, Sallis A, et al. Provision of social norm feedback to high prescribers of antibiotics in general practice: a pragmatic national randomised controlled trial. Lancet 2016;387(10029):1743–52.

28. Olans RD, Nicholas PK, Hanley D, et al. Defining a role for nursing education in staff nurse participation in antimicrobial stewardship. J Contin Educ Nurs 2015; 46(7):318–21.

29. Carter RR, Montpetite MM, Jump RLP. Mixed-methods pilot study to assess perceptions of antimicrobial stewardship in nursing homes. J Am Geriatr Soc 2017; 65(5):1073–8.

30. Toolkit 1. Suspected UTI SBAR Toolkit. Agency for Healthcare Research and Quality Toolkit 2016.

31. Tolg M-SA, Dosa DM, Jump RLP, et al. Antimicrobial stewardship in long-term care facilities: approaches to creating an antibiogram when few bacterial isolates are cultured annually. J Am Med Dir Assoc 2018;19(9):744–7.

32. Fridkin SK, Pack J, Licitra G, et al. Creating reasonable antibiograms for antibiotic stewardship programs in nursing homes: Analysis of 260 facilities in a large geographic region, 2016-2017. Infect Control Hosp Epidemiol 2019;40(8): 839–46.

33. Tolg M-S, Caffrey A, Appaneal H, et al. 1238. A national comparison of antibiograms between veterans affairs long-term care facilities and affiliated hospitals. Open Forum Infect Dis 2018;5(Suppl 1):S376–7.

34. Clinical & Laboratory Standards Institute: CLSI guidelines.

35. Saha SK, Hawes L, Mazza D. Effectiveness of interventions involving pharmacists on antibiotic prescribing by general practitioners: a systematic review and meta-analysis. J Antimicrob Chemother 2019;74(5):1173–81.

36. Loeb M, Bentley DW, Bradley S, et al. Development of minimum criteria for the initiation of antibiotics in residents of long-term-care facilities: results of a consensus conference. Infect Control Hosp Epidemiol 2001;22(2):120–4.

37. High KP, Bradley SF, Gravenstein S, et al. Clinical practice guideline for the evaluation of fever and infection in older adult residents of long-term care facilities: 2008 Update by the infectious diseases society of America. J Am Geriatr Soc 2009;57(3):375–94.

38. Jump RLP, Crnich CJ, Mody L, et al. Infectious diseases in older adults of long-term care facilities: update on approach to diagnosis and management. J Am Geriatr Soc 2018;66(4):789–803.

39. Gupta K, Hooton TM, Naber KG, et al. International clinical practice guidelines for the treatment of acute uncomplicated cystitis and Pyelonephritis in women: a 2010 update by the Infectious Diseases Society of America and the European Society for Microbiology and Infectious Diseases. Clin Infect Dis 2011;52(5): e103–20.

40. Nicolle LE, Gupta K, Bradley SF, et al. Clinical practice guideline for the management of asymptomatic Bacteriuria: 2019 update by the Infectious Diseases Society of America. Clin Infect Dis 2019;68(10):e83–110.

41. Hooton TM, Bradley SF, Cardenas DD, et al. Diagnosis, prevention, and treatment of catheter-associated urinary tract infection in adults: 2009 International Clinical Practice Guidelines from the Infectious Diseases Society of America. Clin Infect Dis 2010;50(5):625–63.

42. McDonald LC, Gerding DN, Johnson S, et al. Clinical practice guidelines for clostridium difficile infection in adults and children: 2017 update by the Infectious Diseases Society of America (IDSA) and Society for Healthcare Epidemiology of America (SHEA). Clin Infect Dis 2018;66(7):987–94.
43. Kalil AC, Metersky ML, Klompas M, et al. Management of adults with hospital-acquired and ventilator-associated pneumonia: 2016 clinical practice guidelines by the Infectious Diseases Society of America and the American Thoracic Society. Clin Infect Dis 2016;63(5):e61–111.
44. Mandell LA, Wunderink RG, Anzueto A, et al. Infectious Diseases Society of America/American Thoracic Society Consensus Guidelines on the management of community-acquired pneumonia in adults. Clin Infect Dis 2007;44(SUPPL. 2):S27–72.
45. Stevens DL, Bisno AL, Chambers HF, et al. Practice guidelines for the diagnosis and management of skin and soft-tissue infections. Clin Infect Dis 2005;41(10): 1373–406.
46. Lipsky BA, Berendt AR, Cornia PB, et al. 2012 Infectious Diseases Society of America clinical practice guideline for the diagnosis and treatment of diabetic foot infections. Clin Infect Dis 2012;54(12):e132–73.
47. Liu C, Bayer A, Cosgrove SE, et al. Clinical practice guidelines by the Infectious Diseases Society of America for the treatment of methicillin-resistant staphylococcus aureus infections in adults and children: executive summary. Clin Infect Dis 2011;52(3):285–92.

Collaborative Antimicrobial Stewardship in the Health Department

Christopher D. Evans, PharmD[a],*, James W.S. Lewis, MD, MPH[b,c,d],*

KEYWORDS

- Antibiotic stewardship • Antibiotic stewardship collaboration • Antibiotic resistance
- Public health • Health care–associated infection prevention

KEY POINTS

- Antibiotic stewardship is fundamentally a collaborative discipline.
- Given the population-level implications of antibiotic resistance and the importance of antibiotic stewardship in prevention of resistance, public health has a vested interest in strengthening antibiotic stewardship efforts.
- State and local public health departments are well positioned to collaborate with a variety of antibiotic stewardship partners within their jurisdictions.
- Collaboration outside of a facility can improve the impact of antibiotic stewardship programs, benefitting the entire community and population at large.

INTRODUCTION

Antibiotic resistance (AR) is an urgent public health threat. The Centers for Disease Control and Prevention (CDC) estimates that each year multidrug-resistant organisms (MDRO) account for more than 2 million illnesses and 23,000 deaths in the United States.[1] Antibiotics are an essential yet shared resource, in that their use, and in particular their overuse, can result in adverse clinical outcomes at the individual patient level and at the population level. Population-level impacts include primarily the spread of resistant pathogens or resistance mechanisms. The development and spread of AR is a complicated and multifaceted problem and therefore collaboration is the cornerstone of any successful antibiotic stewardship program (ASP). As discussed throughout this issue, effective ASPs rely on collaborators within their own

[a] Tennessee Department of Health, Healthcare Associated Infections and Antimicrobial Resistance Program, 710 James Robertson Parkway, Nashville, TN 37243, USA; [b] North Carolina Department of Health and Human Services, Division of Public Health Communicable Disease Branch, 225 North McDowell Street, Raleigh, NC 27603, USA; [c] UNC Gillings School of Global Public Health, 170 Rosenau Hall, CB #7400, 135 Dauer Drive, Chapel Hill, NC 27599-7400, USA; [d] UNC School of Medicine, 321 S Columbia Street, Chapel Hill, NC 27516, USA
* Corresponding authors. 1902 Mail Service Center, Raleigh, NC 27699-1902.
E-mail addresses: christopher.evans@tn.gov (C.D.E.); james.w.lewis@dhhs.nc.gov (J.W.S.L.)

Infect Dis Clin N Am 34 (2020) 145–160
https://doi.org/10.1016/j.idc.2019.10.002
0891-5520/20/© 2019 Elsevier Inc. All rights reserved.

facility (eg, hospital administration, pharmacy, clinicians, nursing, hospital epidemiology and infection prevention [HEIP] programs, clinical microbiology laboratory, the emergency department, information technology, and quality improvement), other acute care hospitals (ACH) within their hospital system, and other types of medical facilities in their system or region (eg, long-term care facilities [LTCF], outpatient clinics, urgent cares, and outpatient pharmacies).[2–6] Finally, public health agencies are important collaborators for any ASP (**Fig. 1**). Given the population-level implications of AR and the importance of antibiotic stewardship (AS) in containment and prevention of resistance, public health has a vested interest in strengthening AS efforts in their jurisdictions. There are opportunities for public health collaboration at all levels including local health departments; state public health programs; and federal public health entities within the Department of Health and Human Services, primarily CDC and its affiliated institutes and offices, such as the National Institutes of Health, Agency for Healthcare Research and Quality, and the Centers for Medicare and Medicaid Services (CMS). This article discusses existing public health stewardship activities and opportunities for collaboration between public health and all of the key partners in the ASP, the potential for improvement and expansion of current activities, and possible new modes of collaboration that could be pursued.

CDC has invested significant resources into promoting AS principles and improving antibiotic use (AU) aside from the core elements framework documents used as benchmarks for ASP requirements. In 2016, the Epidemiology and Laboratory Capacity (ELC) grant expanded its coordinated prevention funding to enhance, in part, AS-related activities by more than $18 million. Primary stewardship activities supported through the ELC grant include the facilitation of core element implementation in all settings across the health care continuum and implementation of targeted projects aimed to improve AU.[7] State and local health departments, as the primary recipients of ELC grant funds, play a critical role as partners in AS. In a framework for public health

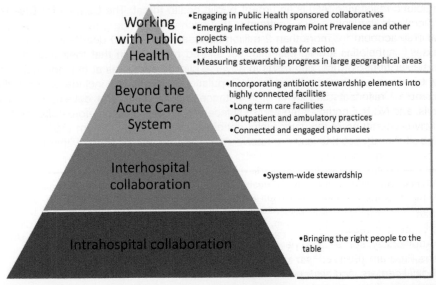

Fig. 1. Antimicrobial stewardship collaborative partnerships. Levels of antimicrobial stewardship collaboration from foundational intrahospital collaboration to regionwide collaboration through collaboration with public health.

departments, CDC outlines activities for implementation of AS at the state, local, or territorial level.[8] These include establishing leadership in the health department, conducting surveillance to understand current stewardship practices and needs, coordinating activities with ongoing quality improvement efforts within the agency and with external public health partners, providing educational tools and resources, developing a communication plan to maintain relationships with partners and organizations, and informing the legislative process. The CDC lists 10 essential public health functions.[9] These have been adapted previously to focus specifically on AS services and are modified here in **Table 1** to include which areas of public health and associated partners would be involved.[10]

GENERAL PUBLIC HEALTH COLLABORATION

Because of the organization of the ELC funding mechanism, many of the AS activities are housed within the state or territory's health care–associated infection (HAI) prevention programs. These programs are the ideal place to identify public health ASP collaborators. State-based HAI contact information is found within CDC's HAI prevention site (https://www.cdc.gov/hai/state-based/index.html).[11] One of the primary ways that public health programs can aid in the advancement of AS efforts is in collaboration with state and jurisdictional partners, including but not limited to state industry organizations for hospitals and LTCFs, hospital improvement innovation networks, and quality improvement networks and organizations. Representatives from these organizations typically serve on advisory groups for state HAI programs, and these groups serve as a starting point for aligning stewardship priorities and activities each organization is undertaking. The state HAI prevention program often serves as a direct link between these organizations and CDC and can facilitate dissemination of CDC-developed tools and resources (eg, core elements for various settings, promotional materials for US Antibiotic Awareness Week [USAAW], and the CDC's AS training modules for providers).[12–17]

State and local public health departments are also well positioned for conducting regional stewardship needs assessments and measuring progress over a specific geographic region. CDC has assessed and published core element attainment progress within the ACH setting at the national level.[18,19] Public health departments have a closer relationship with the facilities within their jurisdiction and can analyze and highlight unique and innovative interventions that facilities have implemented. For example, California's Spotlight on ASPs Project, Georgia and Minnesota's AS Honor Rolls, and North Carolina's Stewardship of Antimicrobial Resources Partners Initiative all give hospital ASPs the opportunity to be publicly highlighted through public facing Web sites and/or social media campaigns.[20–23] The scope of public health programs is broad enough that such assessments and recognition could be performed across multiple health care settings, including long-term care and outpatient settings. Such initiatives are used to track stewardship activities within the state and potentially identify highly effective stewardship strategies when data from these programs are combined with MDRO surveillance data (eg, *Clostridium difficile* infection [CDI] and carbarpenem-resistant Enterobacteriaceae [CRE]).

Additionally, some state health departments are participants in the Emerging Infections Program (EIP). EIP has always promoted strong collaboration with academic medical centers, and several of their projects have significant impact on stewardship at these facilities. EIP performs a periodic point prevalence survey of HAIs in the acute care and long-term care settings. This serves as a unique opportunity for facilities within the 10 EIP epicenters to engage with their public health departments by

Table 1
Antimicrobial stewardship aligns with the 10 essential services of public health

Antimicrobial Stewardship Functions	Relevant Public Health Partners	Relevant Facility-Level ASP Staff/ Partners
Monitor and detect antimicrobial susceptibility patterns and antimicrobial use trends at the national, state, regional, community, and facility levels.	CDC, state health department– HAI/AS staff, QIN-QIO, SLPH	Microbiology, pharmacy, HEIP
Diagnose and investigate concerning patterns and trends in antimicrobial susceptibility across the national, state, regional, community, and facility levels.	CDC, state health department– HAI/AS, local health department communicable disease staff, SLPH	Physicians, HEIP, microbiology
Inform, educate, and empower patients, health care providers, and state survey agencies on appropriate antimicrobial use.	CDC, state health department– HAI/AS staff, local health department communicable disease staff, QIN-QIO, professional organizations, hospital and long-term care associations	Physicians, pharmacists, nurses
Partner with community organizations including but not limited to hospitals, long-term care facilities, health care systems, and patient safety organizations in promoting antimicrobial stewardship strategies across regions, particularly with shared patient populations.	State health department–HAI/AS staff, local health department communicable disease staff, QIN-QIO, hospital and long-term care associations	ASP leaders (physicians/ pharmacists), facility leadership
Identify best practices and policies in antimicrobial stewardship and share them widely.	CDC, state health department– HAI/AS staff	ASP leaders (physicians/ pharmacists)
Advocate for legislation to improve patient safety and protect the public's health by limiting development of resistant infections.	CDC, state health department– HAI/AS staff, hospital associations, and long-term care associations	ASP clinician leaders (physicians/ pharmacists), facility leadership
Link health care facilities with each other to enhance antimicrobial stewardship across regions.	State health department–HAI/AS staff, local health department staff	ASP clinician leaders (physicians/ pharmacists), facility leadership
Ensure competent ASP in health care facilities.	State health department–HAI/AS staff, QIN-QIO	ASP clinician leaders (physicians/ pharmacists)

(continued on next page)

Table 1 (continued)		
Antimicrobial Stewardship Functions	Relevant Public Health Partners	Relevant Facility-Level ASP Staff/Partners
Evaluate and improve ASP in health care facilities.	State health department–HAI/AS staff, QIN-QIO	QI staff, ASP clinician leaders (physicians/pharmacists), HEIP
Research innovative solutions to barriers in antimicrobial stewardship implementation.	CDC, state health department–HAI/AS staff, QIN-QIO	QI staff, ASP clinician leaders (physicians/pharmacists)

Abbreviations: HAI/AS, health care–associated infection/antimicrobial stewardship; QIN-QIO, Quality Improvement Network-Quality Improvement Organization; SLPH, State Laboratory for Public Health,

participating in these point prevalence surveys.[24] The purposes of the surveys are to estimate the prevalence and distribution of HAIs by pathogen and infection site and to estimate the prevalence and appropriateness of AU among US hospitals and LTCFs. The initial hospital point prevalence survey, performed in collaboration with facilities' infection prevention programs and public health personnel, found that 49.9% of hospitalized patients were administered at least one antimicrobial drug; 77% of AU was used for treatment purposes; and use of broad-spectrum antibiotics, such as piperacillin-tazobactam and vancomycin, was common.[25,26] HAI data from the point prevalence survey were used for the development of the CDC Threat Report of 2013, illustrating one example of how facilities' collaboration with public health programs can lead to data for action, an important driver for public health interventions.[1] Multiple other prevention collaborative opportunities are available; details are obtained by reaching out to one's respective state HAI programs. The following sections discuss how public health stewardship staff can interface directly with all of the major ASP team members in a facility.

FACILITY LEADERSHIP

Support and input from C-suite level administrative and quality improvement staff is critical to the development of a successful ASP at the facility level and equally important as ASPs collaborate with public health entities.[12–15,27] The primary roles for hospital administration leaders include but are not limited to writing formal letters of commitment to the ASP mission, requiring ASP activities be included in job descriptions and annual performance reviews, advocating for salary support for ASP team members for their ASP activities, supporting education and training for ASP team members and other hospital staff, and requiring involvement from groups that can support AS activities.[12–15] In a multivariate analysis of hospital core element achievement, O'Leary and colleagues[18] found that written support from administration was the strongest single predictor of a hospital meeting all seven core elements. Financial support greatly augments the capacity and impact an ASP can achieve. Every AS intervention requires three ingredients: (1) time, (2) personnel, and (3) technology. All three of these essential ingredients require money or support from facility administration. Additionally, this administrative endorsement lends weight to recommendations, interventions, educational activities, and projects implemented by ASPs. Involvement in public health stewardship collaboratives, containment and outbreak response, infection control assessments, and facility laboratory interaction with SPHLs (State Public Health Laboratories) all require support from senior hospital leadership to be successful. Facilities having difficulty obtaining leadership support for expanding their stewardship services can provide endorsements from public health when approaching their administration.

An additional method by which public health can advance AS in facilities is by informing the legislative process.[8,10] Health department leadership can educate policy makers on how to advance appropriate AU. This is accomplished through recommendations for stewardship programs in various settings or requiring tracking of AU and prescribing. The process can take significant time and resources, but there are examples of successful implementation. In 2008, California required all ACH to develop processes for improving AU and in 2015, mandated hospitals to implement ASPs that complied with CDC core elements and national guidelines, such as those developed by the Infectious Diseases Society of America (IDSA), the Society of Healthcare Epidemiology of America (SHEA), and the Pediatric Infectious Diseases Society (PIDS).[12,28–30] Following these state laws, California observed an increase in the percentage of ACHs achieving all seven core elements from 59.3% in 2014 to 69.2% in 2015.[28] They also found that hospitals with all infrastructure core elements (ie, leadership, accountability, and drug expertise) were more likely to have all seven core elements achieved than those who did not (unadjusted risk ratio, 2.4; 95% confidence interval, 1.5–3.7).[28] Most states, either through regulation or legislation, have incorporated required reporting of select diseases and/or infectious agents. However, mandated AU reporting remains much more difficult for states. This is in part caused by the time and significant resource burden that must be undergone for ACHs to report AU data into the National Healthcare Safety Network (NHSN).[31] In 2017, Missouri became the first state to pass legislation requiring ACHs to submit data into the NHSN Antibiotic Use and Resistance (AUR) Module.[32,33] More information about the utility of the AUR Module is found in the HEIP section of this article. Tennessee has also implemented a statewide mandate that requires all ACHs to report AU data into NHSN.[34] This regulation for public health reporting was announced in 2018 and will phase different-sized hospitals over several years, with the first requirement for the largest of facilities to be reporting by 2021. Obviously, these processes can have profound impact on what rules and regulations hospitals must follow, and hospital leadership needs to remain informed of these requirements. ASP members, including facility leadership, who collaborate with public health partners can advocate for and help inform the development of such legislation in ways that make it practical to the clinical environments where it will be enforced. State hospital and nursing home associations, with whom public health often has strong ties, commonly work closely with senior facility leadership. Engaging these stakeholders early in the legislative or regulatory process is essential for successful and effective implementation of such requirements. In the Tennessee example described previously, this required early and continued input from members of the Tennessee Hospital Association, the state HAI program, and stewardship and hospital leaders from reporting and nonreporting hospitals.

Finally, the US government has developed an Antimicrobial Resistance Challenge, a way for governments, industries, and other organizations to formally commit to the fight against antimicrobial resistance. To participate, organizations need to show commitment to improving one of the following areas: AU, tracking and reporting, infection prevention, environment and sanitation, and vaccination. Regardless of what area is chosen, senior leadership support is required, and public health is instrumental in spreading the word about this challenge and engaging with organizations to secure their support. Examples of commitments already made are found on the Antimicrobial Resistance Challenge Web site.[35]

PHARMACY, PROVIDERS, NURSING

Physician and pharmacy leaders are the backbone of an effective ASP. CDC, IDSA, SHEA, PIDS, and the Society of Infectious Diseases Pharmacists all recommend ASPs be co-led by a pharmacist and physician.[12,29,30] Pharmacists provide drug expertise and accountability to ASPs and ideally have formalized training in infectious diseases and/or AS. Physicians provide accountability and drug, resistance, and clinical expertise within the ASP and have clinical expertise valued by other providers within the hospital setting.[27] The role of nursing in stewardship activities is garnering increased attention. Nurses have the opportunity to be the front line of AS given their extensive direct patient contact and communication.[36] Further information on the role of nursing in AS is found elsewhere in this issue. Most clinicians and pharmacists are at least tangentially aware of public health work, particularly in outbreak response, but do not understand the breadth and scope of what public health does for the promotion of AS.

Establishing relationships with clinicians and pharmacists in all health care settings is of particular import to public health. This enables smooth communication of public health issues and campaigns (eg, USAAW and CDC Be Antibiotics Aware Campaign).[17,37] These efforts are national educational programs to improve antibiotic prescribing and combat AR. State public health departments play an integral role in communicating information about these campaigns to health care providers within their jurisdictions and can provide promotional materials for each (eg, supportive care prescription pads, appropriate AU posters, and commitment letters). To celebrate USAAW, North Carolina has also hosted a Be Antibiotics Aware Campaign Artwork Competition. Each year, kids from across the state submit artwork addressing appropriate AU; winning pieces are viewed on the North Carolina Antibiotic Resistance Web site and can be ordered free of charge by North Carolina health care facilities that would like to display them.[38] Additionally, CDC has created an interactive World Wide Web–based training on AS that is heavily promoted by state AS programs.[16] This training offers a free continuing education for physicians and other clinicians, pharmacists, and nurses.

To effectively communicate these campaigns and other public health issues to the health care community, the Tennessee HAI program created multiple monthly calls with clinicians across the state, one of which is an antibiotic steward call. It targets pharmacists and physicians in hospital ASPs, and its purpose is to offer advice and expertise on various stewardship interventions from programs already implementing them, discuss relevant stewardship-related issues, report relevant statewide data from the HAI program, and to foster a sense of community among stewardship providers across the state. This call has now been expanded to target stewardship programs in the long-term care setting. It is important for state public health departments to have up-to-date contact information for all stewardship and infection prevention programs across the state. Although most states work diligently to have accurate contacts, ASPs in all types of facilities are encouraged to reach out to their respective state contacts to ensure timely communication of state and national stewardship efforts.[11]

HOSPITAL EPIDEMIOLOGY AND INFECTION PREVENTION

HEIP programs are key partners in any effective ASP.[12] They provide many valuable tools including implementation of appropriate precautions for patients colonized or infected with MDROs, responding to outbreaks in hospital settings (including outbreaks of MDROs), and can provide mentorship and guidance with developing data-based educational materials and presentations for administration regarding the effectiveness of ASPs and for requesting increased resources.[5] Additionally, HEIPs have been reporting HAI data into NHSN for years and have high-level expertise in this activity, which is helpful to ASPs who are interested in reporting AU and AR data into the NHSN AUR module.[31,33,39] Given HEIPs experience working with NHSN they often also have close relationships with state HAI programs and can likely provide an avenue for communication and collaboration with state HAI program staff.

HEIP members of ASPs can facilitate implementing reporting into the NHSN AUR module. The AU option of this module allows reporting of AU measures into NHSN. These data produce the Standardized Antibiotic Administration Ratio, which is a risk-adjusted metric that allows hospitals to compare their AU with other similar systems.[40] Reporting into the AU option requires significant resource allocation and collaboration among HEIP, the ASP team, and information technology. State-based public health programs can offer technical advice as hospitals implement the reporting process. It is possible for hospital system-based ASPs to establish access to these data for all facilities in the system within NHSN through either a data use agreement or through a data rights conferral within the NHSN User Group function. The latter allows view-only access to users to see multiple facilities' AU and HAI data and has been used by state public health departments for HAI surveillance and monitoring ASP's core element implementation in hospitals.[41] The AU option can facilitate the comparison of data from facilities within a system or collaborative, which can subsequently be used to identify trends and catalyze stewardship interventions. The AR option of the AUR module allows reporting of isolate resistance data for a set of common pathogenic bacteria and yeast. As discussed in more detail in the microbiology section, increased uptake of NHSN AR option reporting will provide the potential to generate statewide or even national antibiograms.[33] The data reported into the AU and AR options will allow ASPs to better track the impact of their program activities and can be used to generate data reports, which are helpful in demonstrating impact to administration and demonstrating need for additional resources.

Another pathway for HEIP members of ASPs to collaborate with public health is development of statewide MDRO registries. These registries are a tool used to inform health care facilities on patients with a history of infection or colonization with an MDRO. This efficient communication of a patient's MDRO status allows for timelier implementation of infection-control measures. Currently the only state with an active MDRO registry is Illinois, but CDC is planning to fund at least one more state to develop a similar registry. Likely, registry access will be provided to HEIP program staff in all types of health care settings, allowing for timelier implementation of appropriate precautions with the goal of decreasing the spread of MDROs and ultimately reductions in broad-spectrum AU. HEIP members of ASPs outside of Illinois can work with public health to voice the opinion that this would be a useful containment and stewardship tool. With enough support, it may be possible to obtain state-level funding for MDRO registry development.

MICROBIOLOGY

The microbiology laboratory provides fast, appropriate, and accurate microbiology results to support the application of many AS interventions. The laboratory can implement or advocate for implementation of tests that can further AS efforts by reducing the time to appropriate targeting or discontinuation of antibiotics (eg, procalcitonin testing, rapid molecular testing of respiratory specimens for respiratory viruses, blood culture and cerebrospinal fluid specimens for various pathogens, clinical isolates for specific resistance genes). The laboratory can prioritize processing samples from patients who benefit most from rapid microbiologic data (eg, intensive care and transplant/immunocompromised patients).[5]

In addition to implementing protocols that allow for more rapid antibiotic optimization, they can also institute protocols that improve AU: restricting the antibiotic susceptibility results that are reported (eg, susceptibility test result cascading), and implementation of rejection criteria for clinical specimens with high likelihood of false positivity (eg, poorly collected wound swabs, sputum samples with high levels of epithelial cell contamination, and urine samples with negative urinalyses).[5,42] The laboratory is also essential in development of facility-specific antibiograms. Finally, the laboratory commonly interfaces with public health around disease reporting and surveillance and forwarding concerning isolates to the State Laboratory for Public Health (SLPH), and this relationship can provide an avenue for collaboration between the ASP and public health.[42,43]

Surveillance of MDROs is a large part of state public health programs' responsibilities. As such, they have strong working relationships with their SLPH. This activity can have significant implications on ASPs and the direct patient care in which they are involved. State HAI programs typically monitor the incidence and prevalence of organisms with unique resistance patterns and emerging pathogens or those with significant impact on the health care system. These include, but are not limited to, CRE, carbapenemase-producing CRE, panresistant organisms, vancomycin-resistant *Staphylococcus aureus*/vancomycin-intermediate *S aureus*/methicillin-resistant *S aureus*, *Candida auris*, and others. Although most infectious disease and HAI reporting in the inpatient setting is managed by HEIP teams and the microbiology laboratory, ASPs that are aware of public health reporting requirements can better ensure that these isolates are sent and properly tested by SLPHs, expediting initiation of appropriate antibiotic therapy. In 2016, the CDC also established the Antibiotic Resistance Lab Network, which consists of 56 state and jurisdictional laboratories, seven of which are deemed regional laboratories.[44] These laboratories perform reference characterization and confirmatory antibiotic susceptibility testing of isolates with new and unusual resistance patterns, allow health care facilities access to free shipment for testing of organisms, and offer colonization screening to aid facilities during the containment of resistant pathogens. Additionally, and more specific for stewardship, the Antibiotic Resistance Lab Network is now performing expanded antibiotic susceptibility testing for metallo-β-lactamase-producing Enterobacteriaceae resistant to all Food and Drug Administration–approved drugs. This testing, using technology initially developed for ink-jet printers, enables the laboratory to test for unique combinations of antimicrobials (eg, aztreonam plus avibactam) not otherwise available and helps bridge the gap between new drug approval and the availability of testing methods for hospital laboratories.[45] Moreover, ASPs will be able to directly tailor antibiotic therapy for their patients.

Hospital laboratories are often involved in the development of local susceptibility patterns published routinely as antibiograms. These are often limited to isolates tested at that laboratory. There is interest at the public health level of performing these analyses on a wider geographic area. However, much of the public health reporting of specific organisms has heretofore focused on isolates with unique, novel, or very resistant patterns. Therefore, developing an antibiogram using only isolates submitted to SLPHs would not necessarily give an accurate representation of susceptibility statewide. To overcome this problem, several states have collaborated with individual facility laboratories. In two specific cases out of Virginia and Alaska, laboratories voluntarily shared their facility antibiograms with the state public health department, who then aggregated the data to determine the proportion of isolates of various bacteria that test susceptible to select antibiotics across their respective states/regions.[46,47] Both states performed analyses at the state and various regional levels, because significant differences may exist even among different areas within a given state. With the establishment of NHSN AUR data, state public health departments can also obtain AR data uploaded into the AR option. This also gives the opportunity for states to analyze more granular statewide AR data and not have to go through the process of aggregating multiple facility antibiograms. As a critical mass of facilities begin using the AR option and giving permissions to public health to access their data, these antibiograms will be even more representative of state and regional resistance rates.

QUALITY IMPROVEMENT NETWORKS AND QUALITY IMPROVEMENT ORGANIZATIONS

The CMS supports 14 Quality Improvement Networks–Quality Improvement Organizations (QIN-QIO) who work with health care providers, partners, and beneficiaries on several quality improvement initiatives to improve the care of people with specific health conditions.[48] Through their work, they can help spread best practices to wide geographic regions spanning several states and jurisdictions. Because they have similar priorities and objectives, they often collaborate with state public health departments on projects, including those targeting stewardship and HAI prevention. Recently, select QIN-QIOs have been involved in implementation of core elements in outpatient clinical settings. State public health departments can use their outreach in recruiting practices into this outpatient stewardship collaborative, offer subject matter expertise on core element implementation, and assist in data analysis of core element achievement. Additionally, because they are closely tied to CMS, QIN-QIOs may have access to data to drive stewardship intervention that may not otherwise be readily available to public health. For example, in the previously mentioned collaborative example, the QIN-QIOs had access to prescribing and diagnostic data for Medicaid recipient patient visits. Being able to link outpatient prescribing data to a diagnostic code or indication is useful to determine the appropriateness of antibiotic prescribing, often a difficult metric for stewardship programs to collect and track. Engaging with public health can also help the QIN-QIO to effectively analyze and display these data back to providers in a meaningful way. Other projects that may potentially affect stewardship outcomes in which QIN-QIOs have worked collaboratively with state public health departments include enrolling nursing homes into NHSN for HAI prevention and working to reduce CDI rates through a CDI collaborative. State public health departments can connect organizations and individuals with the QIN-QIOs and inform on what active projects are available for collaboration.

INTERFACILITY COLLABORATION

Once established, a facility's ASP can benefit greatly from collaboration with other facilities within a given system, region, or state. The value of interfacility collaboration cannot be overstated. Not only does it allow the ASP to interact and exchange ideas with other programs, it can potentially allow for peer-to-peer comparison of AS metrics, such as AU and CDI rates. This is of particular import to smaller-sized and critical access hospitals. In the 2015 analysis of core element achievement performed by CDC, 34% of all respondents had a bed size of less than 50, and 18% were designated critical access. Although 66% of all larger hospitals (>200 beds) reported achievement of all seven core elements, only 31% of smaller hospitals had ASPs that achieved all core elements.[18] To incentivize stewardship implementation in critical access hospitals, the Medicare Beneficiary Quality Improvement Program, which supports hospitals through state flex grants, includes implementation of the CDC core elements as a requirement for funding.[49] Approximately 99% of all critical access hospitals participate in this program. To aid smaller facilities in developing their ASPs, CDC developed their Implementation of Antibiotic Stewardship Core Elements at Small and Critical Access Hospitals.[15] The core elements document encourages smaller hospitals to consider enrolling in multihospital, collaborative efforts to improve AU; funding remote consultative or telemedicine services of stewardship experts; and placing stewardship activities into the contractual responsibilities of remote pharmacy services.[15]

Three case examples highlight the importance of engaging experts in the field into an ASP program, even if those experts are not specifically onsite at the hospital. Goff and colleagues[50] highlighted a national AS mentoring program done through the American Society of Health-System Pharmacists where their expert team worked collaboratively with nine hospital sites to expand their ASPs. The Veterans Health Administration implemented an AS initiative, which engaged 250 stewardship champions from 140 hospitals across the country.[51] Finally, Stenehjem and colleagues,[52] at The Intermountain Healthcare System, designed a controlled intervention study to evaluate three potential stewardship strategies across a hospital system administered by the flagship hospitals' ASP. To varying degrees these projects resulted in improvements in facility stewardship metrics, such as stewardship implementation and processes, AU, CDI rates, and readmissions. Collaboratives and telemedicine resources may be difficult for smaller facilities to identify. State and local public health departments can help facilities identify stewardship collaboratives and facilitate collaboration because they are often aware of the activities in their regions. An example of public health departments fostering interfacility ASP collaboration is the North Carolina Stewardship of Antimicrobial Resources Partners initiative. This tiered, recognition-based, incentive program encourages ASP development and to attain the highest tier a facility must indicate that they are willing to mentor another hospital in developing or improving their ASP.[23] Additionally, because most public health stewardship programs are housed within state public health HAI programs, public health ASP staff often have preexisting relationships with infection prevention staff at facilities across the state and with state health care associations and can facilitate collaboration through connecting staff between facilities and organizations.

Interfacility collaboration does not stop at acute care facilities. Collaboration between ACH and LTCFs, emergency departments, urgent care clinics, outpatient clinics, and community-based pharmacies is possible and beneficial. Collaboration between ACH and LTCFs and emergency departments are established practices and have been recommended by AS experts.[13,14,53–61] Although collaboration between ACH ASPs and other outpatient settings and pharmacies is less well established it is certainly possible and has the potential for improvement of AU within the community. State and local public health department AS staff often have working relationships with professional groups, facility staff, and quality improvement organizations (eg, QIN-QIO, Health Improvement and Innovation Network) doing AS-related projects. By forming a working relationship with health departments, facility ASPs can use these connections to foster collaboration.

Finally, health departments may have programs or initiatives that present unique or innovative collaboration opportunities. For instance, the North Carolina Department of Public Health is investigating ways to establish a β-lactam allergy skin testing initiative. If funded, the North Carolina Department of Public Health would target one community-based pharmacist and one primary care provider in each county to award funding for β-lactam allergy skin testing certificate training to provide testing in their facilities. This project would provide an opportunity for ACH in the state to collaborate with the state health department to expand training within their region to other pharmacy and primary care clinic providers through access to local allergy specialists. This is just one example of a potential project that health departments may be interested in developing. Collaboration with one's health department can lead to meaningful collaborations and inform future public health–based projects, such as the ones mentioned in this article.

SUMMARY

AS is fundamentally a collaborative discipline. As outlined in this issue collaboration between multiple departments within a facility is foundational for the establishment of a successful ASP. Collaboration outside of the facility can greatly improve the impact of the ASP and can provide benefit to the entire community, the goal of all public health endeavors. In order for AS efforts to be truly successful, they must reach not only those who most use health care (eg, inpatients, LTCF residents, the chronically ill), but the entire population to foster a culture change around the use of antibiotics. Given their focus of population health and recent increases in funding for AS activities, public health departments are quickly becoming vital partners for ASPs. They will serve as a liaison between state and federal partners and individual facilities. Working with public health can provide access to educational opportunities and materials, facilitate collaboration within and without a facility, and allow the ASP to better inform population-based AS priorities.

DISCLOSURE STATEMENT

Support for this work for both authors was funded by the Epidemiology and Laboratory Capacity Cooperative Agreement.

REFERENCES

1. Centers for Disease Control and Prevention. Antibiotic resistance threats in the United States, 2013. Secondary antibiotic resistance threats in the United States, 2013 2013 April 23. Available at: https://www.cdc.gov/drugresistance/pdf/ar-threats-2013-508.pdf. Accessed December 20, 2018.
2. McEwen SA, Collignon PJ. Antimicrobial resistance: a one health perspective. Microbiol Spectr 2018;6(2). https://doi.org/10.1128/microbiolspec.ARBA-0009-2017.
3. Dingle KE, Didelot X, Quan TP, et al. Effects of control interventions on *Clostridium difficile* infection in England: an observational study. Lancet Infect Dis 2017;17(4): 411–21.
4. Rice LB. Antimicrobial stewardship and antimicrobial resistance. Med Clin North Am 2018;102(5):805–18.
5. Septimus EJ. Antimicrobial resistance: an antimicrobial/diagnostic stewardship and infection prevention approach. Med Clin North Am 2018;102(5):819–29.

6. Tamma PD, Avdic E, Li DX, et al. Association of adverse events with antibiotic use in hospitalized patients. JAMA Intern Med 2017;177(9):1308–15.

7. Centers for Disease Control and Prevention. Epidemiology and Laboratory Capacity for Prevention and Control of Emerging Diseases (ELC). Secondary Epidemiology and Laboratory Capacity for Prevention and Control of Emerging Diseases (ELC) 2019, February 28. Available at: https://www.cdc.gov/ncezid/dpei/epidemiology-laboratory-capacity.html. Accessed March 14, 2019.

8. Centers for Disease Control and Prevention. Antibiotic Stewardship Implementation Framework for Health Departments. Secondary Antibiotic Stewardship Implementation Framework for Health Departments 2017, September 28. Available at: https://www.cdc.gov/antibiotic-use/community/programs-measurement/state-local-activities/framework.html. Accessed December 20, 2018.

9. Centers for Disease Control and Prevention. The Public Health System & the 10 Essential Public Health Services. Secondary The Public Health System & the 10 Essential Public Health Services 2018, June 26. Available at: https://www.cdc.gov/publichealthgateway/publichealthservices/essentialhealthservices.html. Accessed December 20, 2018.

10. Trivedi KK, Pollack LA. The role of public health in antimicrobial stewardship in healthcare. Clin Infect Dis 2014;59(Suppl 3):S101–3.

11. Centers for Disease Control and Prevention. State-based HAI prevention. Secondary state-based HAI prevention 2018, November 12. Available at: https://www.cdc.gov/hai/state-based/index.html. Accessed December 20, 2018.

12. Centers for Disease Control and Prevention. The Core Elements of Hospital Antibiotic Stewardship Programs. Secondary The Core Elements of Hospital Antibiotic Stewardship Programs 2014. Available at: https://www.cdc.gov/antibiotic-use/healthcare/pdfs/core-elements.pdf. Accessed December 20, 2018.

13. Centers for Disease Control and Prevention. The Core Elements of Antibiotic Stewardship for Nursing Homes. Secondary The Core Elements of Antibiotic Stewardship for Nursing Homes 2015. Available at: https://www.cdc.gov/longtermcare/pdfs/core-elements-antibiotic-stewardship.pdf. Accessed December 20, 2018.

14. Centers for Disease Control and Prevention. The Core Elements of Outpatient Antibiotic Stewardship. Secondary The Core Elements of Outpatient Antibiotic Stewardship 2016. Available at: https://www.cdc.gov/antibiotic-use/community/pdfs/16_268900-A_CoreElementsOutpatient_508.pdf. Accessed December 20, 2018.

15. Centers for Disease Control and Prevention. Implementation of Antibiotic Stewardship Core Elements at Small and Critical Access Hospitals. Secondary Implementation of Antibiotic Stewardship Core Elements at Small and Critical Access Hospitals 2017. Available at: https://www.cdc.gov/antibiotic-use/healthcare/pdfs/core-elements-small-critical.pdf. Accessed December 20, 2018.

16. Centers for Disease Control and Prevention. CDC's Antibiotic Stewardship Training Series. Secondary CDC's Antibiotic Stewardship Training Series 2018. Available at: https://www.train.org/cdctrain/training_plan/3697. Accessed January 16, 2019.

17. Centers for Disease Control and Prevention. U.S. Antibiotic Awareness Week (USAAW). Secondary U.S. Antibiotic Awareness Week (USAAW) 2018, October 2. Available at: https://www.cdc.gov/antibiotic-use/week/index.html. Accessed January 16, 2019.

18. O'Leary EN, van Santen KL, Webb AK, et al. Uptake of antibiotic stewardship programs in US acute care hospitals: findings from the 2015 National Healthcare Safety Network Annual Hospital Survey. Clin Infect Dis 2017;65(10):1748–50.

19. Pollack LA, van Santen KL, Weiner LM, et al. Antibiotic stewardship programs in U.S. acute care hospitals: findings from the 2014 National Healthcare Safety Network Annual Hospital Survey. Clin Infect Dis 2016;63(4):443–9.

20. Georgia Department of Public Health. Georgia Honor Roll for Antibiotic Stewardship. Secondary Georgia Honor Roll for Antibiotic Stewardship 2019, January 16. Available at: https://dph.georgia.gov/georgia-honor-roll-antibiotic-stewardship. Accessed January 16, 2019.

21. Minnesota Department of Health. Minnesota Antibiotic Stewardship Honor Rolls. Secondary Minnesota Antibiotic Stewardship Honor Rolls 2019. Available at: https://www.health.state.mn.us/communities/onehealthabx/honor/index.html. Accessed January 16, 2019.

22. California Department of Public Health. California Antimicrobial Stewardship Program Initiative. Secondary California Antimicrobial Stewardship Program Initiative 2018, December 10. Available at: https://www.cdph.ca.gov/Programs/CHCQ/HAI/Pages/CA_AntimicrobialStewardshipProgramInitiative.aspx. Accessed January 16, 2019.

23. North Carolina Division of Public Health. STewardship of Antimicrobial Resources (STAR) Partners Initiative. Secondary STewardship of Antimicrobial Resources (STAR) Partners Initiative 2019, April 22. Available at: https://epi.publichealth.nc.gov/cd/antibiotics/star_partners.html. Accessed December 20, 2018.

24. Centers for Disease Control and Prevention. Emerging Infections Program. Secondary Emerging Infections Program 2018, October 15. Available at: https://www.cdc.gov/ncezid/dpei/eip/index.html. Accessed January 16, 2019.

25. Magill SS, Edwards JR, Bamberg W, et al. Multistate point-prevalence survey of health care-associated infections. N Engl J Med 2014;370(13):1198–208.

26. Magill SS, Edwards JR, Beldavs ZG, et al. Prevalence of antimicrobial use in US acute care hospitals, May-September 2011. JAMA 2014;312(14):1438–46.

27. Ostrowsky B, Banerjee R, Bonomo RA, et al. Infectious diseases physicians: leading the way in antimicrobial stewardship. Clin Infect Dis 2018;66(7):995–1003.

28. Rizzo K, Kealey M, Epson E. Antimicrobial stewardship practices reported by California hospitals following new legislative requirements: analysis of national healthcare safety network annual survey data, 2014-2015. Infect Control Hosp Epidemiol 2017;38(12):1503–5.

29. Barlam TF, Cosgrove SE, Abbo LM, et al. Implementing an antibiotic stewardship program: guidelines by the Infectious Diseases Society of America and the Society for Healthcare Epidemiology of America. Clin Infect Dis 2016;62(10):e51–77.

30. Doernberg SB, Abbo LM, Burdette SD, et al. Essential resources and strategies for antibiotic stewardship programs in the acute care setting. Clin Infect Dis 2018;67(8):1168–74.

31. Centers for Disease Control and Prevention. National Healthcare Safety Network (NHSN). Secondary National Healthcare Safety Network (NHSN) 2017, April 5. Available at: https://www.cdc.gov/nhsn/index.html. Accessed January 16, 2019.

32. Missouri State Senate. SB 579 Modifies provisions relating to infection reporting of health care facilities and telehealth services. Secondary SB 579 Modifies provisions relating to infection reporting of health care facilities and telehealth services 2016, June 8. Available at: http://www.senate.mo.gov/16info/BTS_Web/Bill.aspx?SessionType=R&BillID=22246494. Accessed January 16, 2019.

33. Centers for Disease Control and Prevention. AUR – Surveillance for antimicrobial use and antimicrobial resistance options. Secondary AUR – Surveillance for Antimicrobial Use and Antimicrobial Resistance Options 2019, April 1. Available at:

https://www.cdc.gov/nhsn/training/roadmap/psc/aur.html. Accessed January 16, 2019.

34. Tennessee Department of Health. NHSN Antibiotic Use Reporting. Secondary NHSN Antibiotic Use Reporting 2018. Available at: https://www.tn.gov/content/dam/tn/health/documents/hai/antibiotic-stewardship/AUR_Supplemental_Final_10172018.pdf. Accessed December 20, 2018.

35. Centers for Disease Control and Prevention. The AMR Challenge. Secondary The AMR Challenge 2019, January 31. Available at: https://www.cdc.gov/drugresistance/intl-activities/amr-challenge.html. Accessed January 16, 2019.

36. Sumner S, Forsyth S, Collette-Merrill K, et al. Antibiotic stewardship: The role of clinical nurses and nurse educators. Nurse Educ Today 2018;60:157–60.

37. Centers for Disease Control and Prevention. Be Antibiotics Aware: Smart Use, Best Care. Secondary Be Antibiotics Aware: Smart Use, Best Care 2018, November 9. Available at: https://www.cdc.gov/features/antibioticuse/index.html. Accessed January 16, 2019.

38. North Carolina Division of Public Health. Be Antibiotics Aware: Smart Use, Best Care. Secondary Be Antibiotics Aware: Smart Use, Best Care 2019, April 1. Available at: https://epi.publichealth.nc.gov/cd/antibiotics/campaign.html. Accessed January 16, 2019.

39. Centers for Disease Control and Prevention. Patient Safety Atlas. Secondary Patient Safety Atlas 2019, March 14. Available at: https://www.cdc.gov/hai/data/portal/patient-safety-atlas.html. Accessed December 20, 2018.

40. Centers for Disease Control and Prevention. Antimicrobial Use and Resistance (AUR) Module. Secondary Antimicrobial Use and Resistance (AUR) Module 2019, January. Available at: https://www.cdc.gov/nhsn/PDFs/pscManual/11pscAURcurrent.pdf. Accessed January 16, 2019.

41. Centers for Disease Control and Prevention. DUA FAQs for Health Departments and Facilities. Secondary DUA FAQs for Health Departments and Facilities 2018, March 22. Available at: https://www.cdc.gov/hai/state-resources/dua-faq.html. Accessed January 16, 2019.

42. Bouza E, Munoz P, Burillo A. Role of the clinical microbiology laboratory in antimicrobial stewardship. Med Clin North Am 2018;102(5):883–98.

43. Centers for Disease Control and Prevention. Electronic Laboratory Reporting (ELR) task force overview. Secondary Electronic Laboratory Reporting (ELR) task force overview 2016, August 23. Available at: https://www.cdc.gov/ehrmeaningfuluse/elrtf.html. Accessed January 16, 2019.

44. Centers for Disease Control and Prevention. Lab Capacity: Antibiotic Resistance Laboratory Network (AR Lab Network). Secondary Lab Capacity: Antibiotic Resistance Laboratory Network (AR Lab Network) 2018, September 2018. Available at: https://www.cdc.gov/drugresistance/solutions-initiative/ar-lab-network.html. Accessed January 16, 2019.

45. Centers for Disease Control and Prevention. Pilot Program with HP Accelerates Antibiotic Testing. Secondary Pilot Program with HP Accelerates Antibiotic Testing 2018, August 1. Available at: https://www.cdc.gov/drugresistance/solutions-initiative/innovative-hp-resistance-testing.html. Accessed January 16, 2019.

46. Alaska Division of Public Health. 2015 Alaska State Antibiogram. Secondary 2015 Alaska State Antibiogram 2015. Available at: http://dhss.alaska.gov/dph/Epi/id/SiteAssets/Pages/HAI/default/State%20and%20Regional%20Antibiograms.pdf. Accessed May 10, 2019.

47. Virginia Department of Health. 2017 Virginia State and regional cumulative antibiogram. Secondary 2017 Virginia State and regional cumulative antibiogram

2018, November 9. Available at: http://www.vdh.virginia.gov/content/uploads/sites/13/2018/11/2017-Virginia-State-and-Regional-Cumulative-Antibiogram.pdf. Accessed May 10, 2019.

48. Quality Improvement Organizations. Home Page. Secondary Home Page 2019. Available at: https://qioprogram.org. Accessed May 10, 2019.

49. National Rural Health Resource Center. Medicare Beneficiary Quality Improvement Project (MBQIP). Secondary Medicare Beneficiary Quality Improvement Project (MBQIP) 2019. Available at: https://www.ruralcenter.org/tasc/mbqip. Accessed May 10, 2019.

50. Goff DA, Karam GH, Haines ST. Impact of a national antimicrobial stewardship mentoring program: insights and lessons learned. Am J Health Syst Pharm 2017;74(4):224–31.

51. Kelly AA, Jones MM, Echevarria KL, et al. A report of the efforts of the Veterans Health Administration National Antimicrobial Stewardship Initiative. Infect Control Hosp Epidemiol 2017;38(5):513–20.

52. Stenehjem E, Hersh AL, Buckel WR, et al. Impact of implementing antibiotic stewardship programs in 15 small hospitals: a cluster-randomized intervention. Clin Infect Dis 2018;67(4):525–32.

53. Kullar R, Yang H, Grein J, et al. A roadmap to implementing antimicrobial stewardship principles in long-term care facilities (LTCFs): collaboration between an acute-care hospital and LTCFs. Clin Infect Dis 2018;66(8):1304–12.

54. McElligott M, Welham G, Pop-Vicas A, et al. Antibiotic stewardship in nursing facilities. Infect Dis Clin North Am 2017;31(4):619–38.

55. Lim CJ, Kong DC, Stuart RL. Reducing inappropriate antibiotic prescribing in the residential care setting: current perspectives. Clin Interv Aging 2014;9:165–77.

56. Mistry RD, Newland JG, Gerber JS, et al. Current state of antimicrobial stewardship in children's hospital emergency departments. Infect Control Hosp Epidemiol 2017;38(4):469–75.

57. Grodin L, Conigliaro A, Lee SY, et al. Comparison of UTI antibiograms stratified by ED patient disposition. Am J Emerg Med 2017;35(9):1269–75.

58. Saha D, Patel J, Buckingham D, et al. Urine culture follow-up and antimicrobial stewardship in a pediatric urgent care network. Pediatrics 2017;139(4). https://doi.org/10.1542/peds.2016-2103.

59. May L, Cosgrove S, L'Archeveque M, et al. A call to action for antimicrobial stewardship in the emergency department: approaches and strategies. Ann Emerg Med 2013;62(1):69–77.e2.

60. Zhang X, Rowan N, Pflugeisen BM, et al. Urine culture guided antibiotic interventions: a pharmacist driven antimicrobial stewardship effort in the ED. Am J Emerg Med 2017;35(4):594–8.

61. Baker SN, Acquisto NM, Ashley ED, et al. Pharmacist-managed antimicrobial stewardship program for patients discharged from the emergency department. J Pharm Pract 2012;25(2):190–4.

Moving?

Make sure your subscription moves with you!

To notify us of your new address, find your **Clinics Account Number** (located on your mailing label above your name), and contact customer service at:

Email: journalscustomerservice-usa@elsevier.com

800-654-2452 (subscribers in the U.S. & Canada)
314-447-8871 (subscribers outside of the U.S. & Canada)

Fax number: 314-447-8029

**Elsevier Health Sciences Division
Subscription Customer Service
3251 Riverport Lane
Maryland Heights, MO 63043**

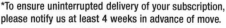

*To ensure uninterrupted delivery of your subscription, please notify us at least 4 weeks in advance of move.

Printed and bound by CPI Group (UK) Ltd, Croydon, CR0 4YY

03/10/2024

01040406-0017